ALZHEIMER'S PATIENTS
IN THE
NURSING HOME:

How Well Do Caregivers
Meet their Needs?

****

ALZHEIMER'S PATIENTS
IN THE
NURSING HOME:

How Well Do Caregivers
Meet their Needs?

Ursula Michelson

****

Library of Congress Number: 2004099611
ISBN :   Hardcover   1-4134-7821-2
                  Softcover   .   1-4134-7820-4

This book was printed in the United States of America.

A portion of the proceeds from the sale of this book will be donated to the Alzheimer's Association, Hudson Valley/Rockland/Westchester, NY Chapter

Grateful acknowledgment is made to the following sources:

1. Mary Lucero for permission to reprint quotations from her Seminars: *Creative Interventions with the Alzheimer's Patient*, Videotapes, copyright© 1992 by Geriatric Resources, Inc., Winter Park, Florida.

2. The Crisis Prevention Institute, Inc. for permission to reprint quotations from their *Participant Workbook for the* Nonviolent Crisis Intervention® *Training Program*, Brookfield, WI: Crisis Prevention Institute, Inc., 2005

Author Photo: Sean Scott Smith

To order additional copies of this book, contact:
Xlibris Corporation
1-888-795-4274
www.Xlibris.com
Orders@Xlibris.com
25321

In memory of
Jess Maverick McNeel Gordon
who was instrumental in making this book possible.
In his honor, and in consideration of the suffering that
characterized much of his life, it is hoped that this book
will result in the alleviation of some measure of suffering
in the lives of others.

Acknowledgments

My most heartfelt gratitude and thanks to my friend and mentor, Laura Gordon Georgakakos, who encouraged and inspired me to write about my experiences with Alzheimer's patients in the nursing home. Her generosity and guidance were a constant throughout the preparation of the manuscript. Her editorial skills have been invaluable in the creation of this book. Without her continued enthusiasm and support for this project, it would never have come to fruition.

Thank you to Meg Boyce, director of programs and service of the Alzheimer's Association, Hudson Valley, Rockland, Westchester, New York Chapter, for her careful reading of the manuscript and her thoughtful comments and suggestions.

Thank you to Julie Torman, MD, gastroenterologist, and Thaddeus Wandel, MD, ophthalmologist, who gave of their valuable time to vet the medical information conveyed in the chapters that pertain to their respective specialties.

The encouragement and feedback provided by family and friends are deeply appreciated. Thank you, Sheilah Beckett, Gwen Erdlitz, Helen Johnson, and Linda McCreery.

Thank you to my daughters, Robin Nourie and Karen Torsiello, and to their spouses, Rich Nourie and Mario Torsiello. Your love sustained me during the years this book evolved to its final form.

Thank you to my editors Mark Ranel Lambo and Kevin Desabelle at Xlibris for their careful editing of the manuscript.

Disclosure

All the names of persons mentioned in this book, as well as the names of the nursing homes and their locations, and certain other identifying information, have been changed for the following reasons:

a. As a provider of mental health services to nursing home residents, I am ethically and legally bound to protect the confidentiality and privacy of all the clients who received these services.

b. While I feel strongly that the information conveyed in this book, regarding the distressing experiences the Alzheimer's residents were subjected to, need to be brought to the attention of the public, it is not my intention to place blame on individual caregivers or on any of the nursing homes in which the events related in this book took place. These nursing homes are by no means the only facilities that fail to provide quality care for Alzheimer's residents. Failures of many nursing homes in the United States to provide quality care is a serious long-standing problem, as has been reported by State Inspectors for many years.

The conversations with nursing home residents and staff have been recorded as best I can recall. In some instances, they may not be the exact words in which they occurred, however, they are faithful to the essence of verbal exchanges between myself and others. In many instances it was easy to recall the exact words used by the Alzheimer's residents, because much of what they communicated was so memorable, that to this day, I could recite their words in my sleep.

Ursula Michelson

*I'm going to sleep now. You better leave me alone or
I'm going to kill you.*

—Sarah

Chapter 1

At 8:00 AM on a Tuesday morning, I walked into the Oak Terrace Nursing Home. Before I had crossed the length of the elegantly appointed reception area on my way to the South Unit, the administrator, John Weber, rushed up to me and exclaimed, "I'm so glad you are here, Ursula, we have a crisis on our hand and need your help."

It was the second day of my new job as coordinator of a mental health service for nursing-home residents, and I had not yet had time to get to know the facility, the staff, or the residents.

As we rushed down the long hallway toward the Alzheimer's unit, Mr. Weber filled me in on the particulars of this crisis: The previous evening, close to the dinner hour, Sarah, one of the Alzheimer's residents, had wandered into another resident's room and refused to come out. Several of the nurses and CNAs (certified nursing assistants) pleaded with her for cooperation—all to no avail. Sarah refused to budge.

Eventually, one of the CNAs marched into the room, took Sarah firmly by the arm, and attempted to escort her out, telling her she needed to go to the dining room to eat. Sarah was furious. She assaulted the aide, kicking, and scratching her, and then shoved her out the door.

By now, three shifts of caregivers had attempted to coax Sarah out of the room without success. She had wedged a heavy lounge chair between the wall and the door of the room so that the door could only be opened a few inches. She had spent the night and was, as of this moment, still in there.

As I listened to the administrator explain the situation, it flashed through my mind that the success or failure of my intervention with Sarah would affect my credibility with this nursing home staff forever after. Although my staff and I had met with a group of the caregivers at this facility several days ago, to introduce ourselves and to explain the goals and objectives of the Mental Health Nursing Home Program, I was still a virtual stranger here. I had hoped to establish rapport and mutual respect with the caregivers, as I believed this to be essential for effective communication with everyone involved in the care of the residents who would become our clients.

Just the day before we had been given the list of names of those residents who had been recommended and approved by their physicians to participate in our service. We were just beginning to get to know these residents and to work up their assessments. I had expected that we would be fully occupied with that process for the next several days. And although crisis intervention was one of the services included in our program, I had not anticipated that I would be called on so soon for such intervention. My tension mounted as we arrived at the room Sarah occupied.

I did not yet know anything about this resident, except that she had early-onset Alzheimer's disease, was in her late fifties, physically strong and quick to become abusive with caregivers. Mr. Weber characterized her as "probably the most challenging resident we have." He said that some of the caregivers were intimidated by Sarah, and quite a few of them had received bruises or even a black eye during their encounters with her.

Several nurses and aides were standing in front of the room Sarah had appropriated the night before. One of them had her head close to the narrow opening of the door, and I heard her admonishing the resident in a stern voice. "Sarah, push that chair away from the door, at once and come out! We have had enough of this nonsense. If you don't come out now, you won't get any breakfast."

I couldn't believe my ears. I wondered if the speaker actually expected Sarah to comply.

Mr. Weber introduced me and told the assembled nurses and CNAs, most of whom I had not met before, that he had asked me to try and get Sarah out of that room. He then asked the staff to cooperate and assist me as needed.

From the way some of the staff looked me over, I could tell that they resented my intrusion into what they considered to be their territory. I did not feel comfortable having to direct any requests to them, but it was necessary to put personal feelings aside and to concentrate on what needed to be done.

I asked everyone to leave the immediate area in front of the room Sarah occupied to give me time alone with her. After everyone had pulled back, I waited a few moments and then put my face to the opening of the doorway and got my first glimpse of her. She had large gray eyes, a round unlined face framed by short-cropped gray hair. She was of sturdy build, and she looked younger than most people her age. She was seated upright on the bed, humming to herself, but kept a watchful eye at the narrow opening at the door.

"Good morning, Sarah." I called out to her and smiled.

She frowned. "Who are you?" she asked.

"My name is Ursula."

Sarah continued to frown. "What do you want?" she asked suspiciously.

"Oh, I don't want anything," I assured her. "I just wanted to say hello. You see I'm new here. I don't know anybody. I was hoping to get to know you. I thought maybe we could be friends." I waited for her reaction. I had deliberately paused between each sentence in order to give her time to process the information.

Slowly her frown was replaced by a smile, "That would be nice. I could use a friend," she said.

This was more encouraging than I had hoped. I wondered if I

could push my luck. "Sarah," I asked, "would it be OK if I came in to visit with you for a while?"

She thought that over for a moment, then nodded her head, "Sure," she said, "that's all right."

"But Sarah," I told her, "I can't open the door. I think it's stuck. Would you help me open it, please?"

Sarah got off the bed, moved the chair, and opened the door wide. As I stepped across the threshold, she climbed back onto the bed while I remained standing just inside the doorway, which was about four feet from the bed. We studied each other. I was keenly aware of the importance of giving her time to feel comfortable with me.

Although Sarah had been friendly enough so far, her acceptance of me was still tentative. I sensed that she was very much on her guard. She did not yet entirely trust that my intentions were friendly.

She had taken off all her clothes except her bra and panties. It was cold in the room and she had pulled the thin blanket on the bed up to cover her legs. She was sitting up rigidly with her arms wrapped around herself.

"Would you like another blanket?" I asked her.

"That would be nice," she replied

I stuck my head into the hallway and asked one of the caregivers, who were hovering nearby, to bring me a blanket. I cautioned them to stay out of sight, but close enough to assist if anything else was needed.

The blanket was promptly brought and I tucked it gently around Sarah. "Oh," she commented, "that feels so much better. You are so nice."

I asked her if she would like breakfast. "Yes, please," she replied cheerfully.

I stuck my head out the door once more and asked for Sarah's breakfast tray. As we waited for it, I engaged her in conversation, and she readily answered my questions about herself and her family. She told me about her "daddy" who was a police officer, and about her mother who played the piano and sang in the church choir. When asked if she was married, she replied in the affirmative and stated her husband's name was Harry. When I asked her if she had children, she looked puzzled for a moment and stared into space. Then her faced brightened and she replied, "I have two sisters, Maureen and Regina and a brother named Harry."

I found out later, when I perused Sarah's personal history in her medical chart, that she had a daughter and a son and that her husband's name was Robert. The nurses told me that Sarah's family came to visit with her regularly, but that she recognized neither her husband nor her children. All her memories appeared to pertain to her life prior to adulthood.

When her breakfast tray arrived, I placed it on the tray table by the bed, adjusting it to the proper height for Sarah. She ate and drank everything on her tray, then pushed it back and looked at me expectantly.

"Sarah," I told her, "It's a beautiful day. I'm going for a walk in the garden. Would you like to come?"

"Yes, I would love that!" she said, and immediately got off the bed.

She allowed me to help her get dressed, and left the room with me without a backward glance. She agreed just as readily to my suggestion that she might want to dress in a warmer outfit, as it was still cool outside and "we want to be comfortable on our walk."

After we got to her room, she agreed to wash her hands and face, and to brush her teeth. She even permitted me to comb her hair. All of this was done without protest. I took her out for a walk around the facility's grounds, and after half an hour she agreed to come inside to attend the morning's recreation program, which was about to begin in the dining room.

Later that day, I met with the caregiving staff that had been involved in the crisis. The purpose of the meeting, which had been arranged by Mr. Weber, the administrator, was to discuss how the problem with Sarah had escalated to the degree that it had, and why my intervention had been successful so quickly. Mr. Weber wanted me to teach the staff the skills and strategies I had used in my interactions with Sarah.

At first, as I had expected, I encountered a certain amount of hostility and defensiveness from the staff, especially from Kelly, the CNA, who had initially attempted to get Sarah out of the room by taking her arm, an action that had backfired and earned her a few bruises.

"All I did was tell Sarah that this was not her room and that she couldn't stay there," Kelly explained. "When she refused to pay any attention to me, I took hold of her arm and started to walk her toward the door. I wasn't rough with her, just firm. That's when she scratched and kicked me."

Kelly fell silent, and Elsa, another aide, explained what happened next.

"I was just walking past the room when I saw that Kelly was having trouble with Sarah, so I called down the hall to the nurses' station to let them know we needed help. Sandy and Maria came down right away, and we all tried to get Sarah to leave Mildred's room. But by now she was in a real rage, swinging and punching at anyone who came near her."

Maria broke in, "I told the girls that we needed to back off—give Sarah time to cool down. So we all left the room, hoping that maybe she would come out by herself.

"Dinnertime was approaching," continued Maria, "and Sarah still hadn't budged from Mildred's room, I walked down the hall again. I didn't go into the room, I just stuck my head in the door and said, 'Sarah, it's time to go to the dining room to eat.'

"She just looked at me angrily and yelled, 'Get away from that door. I'm not going!'

"We waited a while. I sent one of the girls down every ten minutes for the next half hour to ask Sarah to come to the dining room."

"Yes," continued Ellie, "and every time she saw one of us, she slammed the door and refused to cooperate."

"It was getting late, so we decided to bring in her dinner tray, hoping that eating might calm her down," said Sandy, "but even that didn't do any good. I went into the room after she had finished eating, and I said, 'Sarah, it's bedtime. Wouldn't you like to sleep in your own room, in your own bed?' She got mad allover again and threw her dinner tray at me.

"So I said, 'OK, OK, Sarah. It's all right,' and I just gathered up the mess as fast as I could, and backed out of the room with it."

Maria, the nursing supervisor, took up the narrative again. "We tried several more times to talk Sarah into leaving Mildred's room. We even tried to bribe her with a promise of ice cream. Sarah loves chocolate ice cream. But even that didn't tempt her to come out."

"By nine o'clock she had taken her clothes off, climbed into Mildred's bed, and told us, "I'm going to sleep now. You better leave me alone or I'm going to kill you.""

"You've got to understand," broke in Kelly, "that all this time Mildred was very upset. She cried inconsolably because she couldn't go to her room. So we had more than one hysterical resident on our hands."

"We tried one more time to get Sarah out of Mildred's room," resumed Maria. "I took Mildred, who was still crying, with me. I held her hand as we approached her room. We didn't go in, but I let Sarah see her, because Sarah and Mildred usually get along well. I had hoped that if Sarah could see how unhappy Mildred was, she would give up her room to her. Well, that turned out to be the worst idea I had.

"When Mildred saw Sarah in her bed, she began to howl, 'That's my bed, get out!' Sarah got off the bed, and for one moment we all believed she was actually going to leave the room, as she walked toward the door. Instead she quickly slammed the door in our faces, and when we tried to open it, we couldn't. Sarah had wedged Mildred's armchair between the wall and the door. The door opened only wide enough to provide a view of part of the bed, and Sarah was back in it, pulling the blanket up to her chin."

Sandy continued, "You can't imagine Mildred's outrage. It took us nearly an hour to calm her down. But Mildred is a more reasonable person than Sarah, and eventually, she agreed to sleep in another room."

"By the time the night shift arrived at eleven, both Mildred and Sarah were asleep, and we were exhausted."

Now Laura took over. "When we came on duty at seven this morning, the night shift filled us in on the situation, and since we found Sarah to be awake when we went to check on her, we too tried to get her to come out of Mildred's room. But as you know, we didn't get anywhere either."

"So, tell us, Ursula," questioned Anna, "what did you do to get Sarah out of that room without a fight?"

Everyone looked at me expectantly, but not without a certain amount of resentment. Hoping to gain some goodwill, I said, "First of all, I was a new face for Sarah, and I was not wearing a uniform. So she didn't associate me with staff. Remember, by the time I came along Sarah was pretty angry at all of you."

As diplomatically as I could, I explained to them why their approaches and interactions with Sarah had been doomed to failure.

First of all, telling Sarah that this was not her room, and that was why she had to get out had no meaning for her. An Alzheimer's patient with the severity of cognitive impairment Sarah had suffered can no longer relate to the concept of ownership (i.e., this is not *your* room; it belongs to someone else, etc.).

Second, anytime you tell someone like Sarah that they are not allowed to do something, they feel threatened, and become defensive.

Third, putting one's hands on the person, even when done gently and with good intentions, implies use of force, which triggers fears and leads to greater resistance than mere words. It compels the person to lash out in self-defense.

Fourth, adding other people to the situation makes the person feel outnumbered, powerless. In most cases it will result in a panic reaction. Now the person is totally out of control and will lash out at anyone who comes close.

My approach in resolving the impasse with Sarah included the following strategies:

- I made no demands on Sarah. I never mentioned that she was in the wrong room.
- I deliberately made our encounter a pleasant one. Everything I said and did conveyed my respect and my concern for her comfort. I gave her as much control of the situation as possible.
- I was careful not to invade her private space. In the beginning of my approach to her, I deliberately kept what I knew to be a reasonable distance from her.
- I gave her time to study me and to process the information I conveyed to her.
- I asked her permission each time I wanted to move closer to her, even when I wanted to do something for her comfort, such as getting her an extra blanket or bringing her breakfast.
- When I invited her to come for a walk with me, to go to her room, to change her clothes, etc., I gave her the choice to say no.
- I validated her communication to me. I made her feel valued by my approach, and this resulted in trust and rapport between us. I do believe it was crucial that only one person interacted with Sarah to resolve the standoff.

As fraught with tension as the meeting with the caregivers had been at the beginning, it did conclude on a positive note. I acknowledged that it must be very difficult and frustrating for the caregivers to have to spend so much time with one resident, when there are so many others who need attention and care.

Since few of those present had met me prior to my appearance that morning, and none of them knew much about me, I used this opportunity to tell them about my past experience in working with mental patients at a psychiatric hospital and subsequently with Alzheimer's patients at an all-Alzheimer's facility. I talked about our program and our mission to reduce the mental anguish and depression of our clients at the nursing home.

I expressed the hope that our work with these residents would also reduce the amount of time they, as caregivers, would have to spend with residents like Sarah, who tended to act out when they experienced emotional distress.

I assured them that we would be a daily presence at Oak Terrace. Three of the mental health nursing home specialists had already been assigned to work at this facility. I told them that crisis intervention was included in the services we provided, and they should feel free to call upon us to assist them as needed.

I then pointed out that we, in turn, would appreciate the caregivers' input regarding our clients. "Since you spend more time with your residents than anyone else, you know their problems and concerns better than anyone," I told them. "It will be of immense help to us if you will allow us to consult with you and are willing to share with us your concerns for your residents."

We had made a good beginning in establishing trust and rapport between us. In time, we came to appreciate each other's work and our daily interactions and communications on behalf of the residents were beneficial to all of us, especially to the residents we served.

I was, however, surprised that the nurses and the CNAs at the Oak Terrace had such poor skills in their interactions with Alzheimer's residents. After all, according to statistics, between 60 and 80 percent of all nursing-home residents in the United States are suffering from dementia—the majority of them from dementia of the Alzheimer's type.

We did not know it at the time, but the crisis intervention with Sarah was only the first of many such interventions my staff and I provided during the next several years. In many instances, as was the case with Sarah, the crisis resulted from caregivers' lack of education about Alzheimer's disease. This was not only the case at the Oak Terrace but at all the other facilities served by the Mental Health Nursing Home Program in this community.

What would become of me should my condition deteriorate? Would I be cared for, treated with kindness and concern? Or would I be an unwelcome and resented burden, a source of contention, or worse, deemed nonexistent? Would I be permitted to retain a degree of dignity and quality of life, or would I be considered human refuse, without merit, without feelings?

—Diana Friel McGowin
Living in the Labyrinth[1]

Chapter 2

Alzheimer's disease was first identified and differentiated from other types of dementia (those caused by strokes, brain injury, accident, or by other diseases) in 1906, by Alois Alzheimer, a German physician. It is a progressive, degenerative disease that to date is irreversible and ultimately fatal.

The onset of AD is insidious. Short-term memory loss and forgetfulness are usually the first symptoms to appear. The person may repeat the same question, or tell the same story over and over, within minutes, without being consciously aware of having done so. Other gaps in the memory system follow, such as forgetting words during conversation, forgetting names of familiar persons and places, forgetting appointments, and misplacing things. Such incidents may be the first indication to the person's family and friends that there is a problem.

As these gaps in the person's memory increase, they begin to interfere with his/her activities of daily living, including job performance and the discharge of other duties and responsibilities.

Eventually tasks that once were performed with ease (keeping a checkbook, cooking a meal, etc.), become difficult, then impossible to perform. As these episodes increase, the person becomes frightened, insecure, and embarrassed. Self-esteem plummets. The person spends much time seeking to cover up for these lapses or to compensate for them in ingenious ways.

Concurrently, or some time later, the patient begins to experience episodes of confusion and disorientation. These can be truly terrifying. Picture yourself going to your local supermarket, something you have been doing several times per week for many years. Suddenly the place looks totally unfamiliar to you. You don't know where you are, or how you got there. Worst of all, you don't remember where you live, or how to get home. Imagine your feelings of terror if this happened to you.

Many people experience such episodes in the early stages of Alzheimer's. At first, these episodes may happen only occasionally and the person may continue to function reasonably well. The next time she goes to the supermarket, she may have no problem at all in doing the shopping and finding the way home. But a week or several weeks later, the confusion and disorientation may strike again, perhaps in another location, at work or while driving on a highway.

As the gaps in memory, confusions, and disorientation and the difficulties in managing daily responsibilities increase, the afflicted person's emotional distress becomes more acute as well.

Alzheimer's is a very isolating disease. Many patients tend to withdraw from social contact with family and friends in an attempt to hide the extent of their dysfunction. Depression and anxiety can become overwhelming.

One need only read Diana Friel McGowin's book, *Living in the Labyrinth: A Personal Journey Through the Maze of Alzheimer's*,[2] to understand how much emotional distress is experienced by a person in the early stages of AD.

As the disease progresses, the person will suffer severe cognitive impairment that will interfere with the ability to comprehend complex concepts, understand and process information, and make rational judgments and appropriate decisions.

In most cases, families and friends of the afflicted will notice significant changes in his/her personality, mood, and behavior. The person tends to be more irritable and may express paranoid ideation, accusing those around him of stealing or hiding from him items he has misplaced.

Sooner or later, the ability to comprehend and use language will become more seriously impaired, and the person's ability to use verbal communication declines, incrementally, until his/her verbal expressions are reduced to babble.

Eventually, the person will lose awareness that he is not functioning as well as he once did and is then no longer concerned with what has happened to him.

However, this does not mean that he now ceases to suffer emotional distress. On the contrary, having lost the ability to orient himself in his surroundings, to recognize others who once were familiar to him, and to understand what is being communicated to him, he feels even more isolated, insecure, and frightened.

Even as his thought processes become totally disorganized, he continues to experience the full range of emotions (both positive and negative). How he feels at any given moment depends on a complex set of circumstances and is influenced by his physical environment, his level of comfort in it, and how his caregivers and others interact with him—be they family, friends, or professional caregivers.

To complicate matters further, once the person has lost the ability to accurately process and organize the stimuli that surrounds him—all that he sees, hears, and experiences—his perceptions tend to be based on misperceptions and misinterpretation. At the same time his ability to use language and to communicate his needs/ wants to others are greatly diminished or lost entirely.

All of the these factors cause the patient acute emotional distress and frustration, feelings that frequently lead to inappropriate behaviors as his sole means to express these feelings. Such behaviors may include resistance to care, attempts to elope, verbal and/or physical abuse toward others, etc.

As if in compensation for the loss of cognitive processes, the person becomes more highly sensory oriented, and his primary focus shifts to what feels safe and comfortable—what feels good. He may engage in self-stimulation, or in other repetitive behaviors, such as rummaging, picking at his clothes, and hoarding things.

He may be putting things in his mouth, sucking or chewing them, whether or not they are edible. He may pace continuously, to the point of exhaustion, unable to stop, and caregivers have to step in to rescue him from this activity.

It has often been said that Alzheimer's patients engage in purposeless activities, but most experienced caregivers have come to agree that there is a purpose to the many and varied activities these patients pursue. They appear to be always searching for someone or something that looks familiar and that they can relate to—someone or something that will provide reassurance in a world that has become increasingly unrecognizable to them.

Whereas in the earlier stages of AD the afflicted person tends to isolate himself from social situations, he now spends much time seeking companionship, a friend—a buddy. Mary Lucero,[3] a gerontologist and lecturer on AD, has characterized Alzheimer's patients in the middle stages of the disease as "social butterflies," a very apt description.

In the nursing homes one often encounters two Alzheimer's patients walking through the facility holding hands, cheerfully engaged in conversation only they can understand. One also frequently sees a resident who follows a nurse or a visitor around, even introducing that person as his "best friend," or a relative.

Many Alzheimer's patients in the middle stages of the disease are very tolerant, even solicitous and nurturing with their peers. And they are highly responsive to attention and affection from anyone willing to provide these.

Sadly, new disabilities continue to make their appearance. Changes in posture, gait, and balance begin to occur. The patient may become unsteady on his feet. He may begin to lean to one side or the other, depending on which side of his brain the destruction of brain cells predominates. At this point, the person becomes highly vulnerable to falls and injuries.

There are many voluntary bodily functions which, once mastered (usually during the first eighteen months of life), we thereafter perform without conscious thought, such as sitting down, standing up, walking, running, picking up food with a spoon or fork, and bringing it to one's mouth. Coordination of these functions is controlled by the cerebellum, which signals the appropriate set of muscles to move as we wish. When this motor control is no longer functioning, the patient's muscles fail to receive these signals, and he needs a caregiver's assistance to jump-start him in walking or in performing any of the other movements formerly activated by the brain.

Once the brain damage has reached that stage of severity, the patient is moving into the final stages of the disease, during which he becomes bedridden and is as helpless as an infant in its first weeks of life. He can no longer hold up his head or feed himself and will most likely begin to have difficulty swallowing his food as his swallowing reflex begins to deteriorate. At this point, all his food must be pureed to reduce the risk of choking or aspirating food particles into his lungs.

He may survive in that state for an unpredictably long time, but eventually the disease reaches the brain stem, which controls and regulates the body's involuntary function of such organs as the heart, liver, lungs, and kidneys, and the metabolic processes involved in digesting nourishment. At this point death is imminent.

It is not yet known why, but there is significant variation in how long it takes for a person to move from mild impairment to the kind of massive brain damage that places him into the midrange and, subsequently, into the final stage of the disease. All of these losses of specific brain function do not occur within the same time frame for all Alzheimer's patients. Patients can survive with this disease for as long as twenty years after onset, although many of them succumb to other diseases long before Alzheimer's disease has run its course.

Scientists now believe that there are several kinds of dementia of the Alzheimer's type. It is generally true that in patients with early onset of AD (before age sixty-two), the disease progresses more rapidly than it does in those with later onset. Statistically, most patients with early onset have significantly shorter life spans.

However, once a diagnosis of Alzheimer's has been made, it is not so much fear of dying as it is fear of living with the disease that concerns the patients and their families.

There is no doubt that every person afflicted with AD experiences acute emotional distress during the course of this terrible disease. These patients need and deserve all the support and TLC their caregivers can render them.

Those who believe that Alzheimer's patients do not suffer emotional distress, "because they don't know what is happening to them"—and there are still many such people, including caregivers—could not be more mistaken.

The effects of the disease are emotionally devastating to the patient. Anxiety, depression, fear, despair, and panic accompany him on his journey through AD as he struggles to cope with the gradually increasing losses of life skills that most of us take for granted. These are the skills that human beings need in order to make sense of the world they inhabit and to function adequately.

Many caregivers fail to understand that when an Alzheimer's patient begins to exhibit inappropriate behaviors, it is a signal that he is in emotional distress and/or physical discomfort and needs attention. It is the caregiver's approach and his or her level of skill in interacting with such residents that determines the outcome of the situation. If they fail to respond to a distraught resident with patience, kindness, and reassurance, if they do not have the skills to help the person to calm down and to restore his emotional comfort, then the caregiver's behavior will only escalate the resident's distress and may provoke a panic reaction, or as it is called, a catastrophic outburst.

There are long-term care facilities where the physical environment and the caregiving routines have been adapted to the special care needs of the Alzheimer's residents, and where staff have been trained to communicate appropriately with them. In such facilities there are far fewer catastrophic outbursts and other problem behaviors, and residents are generally more content. Serious problems arise in those facilities in which management has ignored the need for their caregiving staff to be educated in Alzheimer's disease and in caregiving strategies for this resident population.

I well remember my own ignorance about Alzheimer's disease the first time I came face to face with someone who had been diagnosed with it. At the time, I was the director of the recreation department of a private psychiatric hospital in New York, when a new patient was admitted. He was a fifty-six-year-old male with early-onset AD. This man, a former diplomat at UN headquarters in New York, was already severely cognitively impaired.

According to his wife, he had been fluent in five languages prior to his illness, but now had lost all verbal abilities, and no longer recognized his wife or his children. He had been brought to our facility for evaluation due to his propensity for violent outbursts, which included striking his wife and generally exhibiting out-of-control behaviors. He was in a highly agitated state upon admission.

For the three-and-a-half years since he had been diagnosed with AD, he had been cared for at home, around-the-clock, by professional caregivers. In the past several months, however, his behavior had become increasingly erratic and violent, and, his wife explained, it had become impossible to find caregivers willing to stay and care for him.

Within days of his arrival at the hospital, Mr. D. responded to the psychotropic medication prescribed for him. After his mood and behavior had stabilized, he was brought to the recreation department several hours each day.

He proved to be a challenge both for me and for my staff which we did not meet successfully. To this day, I remember how powerless I felt to do anything of therapeutic value for this patient.

Mr. D. did not respond to any of our attempts to gain his attention and to establish some kind of interaction that would be meaningful for him. We tried to engage him in some very simple activities, but he showed no interest.

Some of the other patients initially tried to befriend him, talk to him, and show him their projects, but after they failed to elicit even the most minimal response, they gave up and ignored him.

Day after day Mr. D. sat in one of the big easy chairs and stared into space. When his wife visited him, there was no change in his expression, and he remained as indifferent to her as he was to everyone else. In retrospect, I believe that he was likely overmedicated, which would account, at least in part, for his apathy. Fortunately for him, within a short time he was transferred to a more appropriate facility.

After this single encounter with an Alzheimer's patient, I came to the erroneous conclusion that nothing could be done to improve the quality of life for a person with this disease. I too believed that Alzheimer's patients did not suffer emotionally since they did not have any awareness of what was happening to them. Years would pass before I learned just how wrong I was.

---

1. Diana Friel McGowin, *Living in the Labyrinth: A Personal Journey Through the Maze of Alzheimer's,* (New York: Elder Books, 1993), 105.
2. ibid.
3. Mary Lucero, Lecturer: *Creative Interventions with the Alzheimer's Patient*, Videotape Lecture (Winter Park, Florida: Geriatric Resources, Inc., 1992).

I'm so glad you could come! This is going to be a wonderful party.
All my friends are here.

—Harriet

Chapter 3

More than a decade passed before Alzheimer's disease was brought to my attention once more. By 1992, I had relocated to Florida and was searching for a job. But at that time and place jobs were scarce, especially in the field of mental health. Through an acquaintance, I was offered a part-time position in the recreation department of a long-term care facility for Alzheimer's patients called Magnolia Manor.

At first, I did not know how to respond to this offer. I needed a job desperately, even if it was only part-time, but I had grave doubts as to whether I would feel comfortable working with this particular population of patients. I knew nothing about Alzheimer's beyond the fact that it was an incurable progressive disease that caused dementia. And I couldn't help but recall my frustrating experience with Mr. D. all those years before, and my failure to do anything constructive for him. I shared my misgivings with Alicia, the director of Magnolia Manor's recreation department.

"Don't worry about that," she said. "This is not so different from working with psychiatric patients, which you have done for so many years. I just know you'll be great for this job."

I did not share her confidence, but rather than accept or decline the offer, I asked permission to spend a day at the facility to familiarize myself with the residents, as well as with the duties and

29

responsibilities the job entailed. By the end of the day I would know whether the job was right for me and, more importantly, whether I was the right person to work with these special residents. Alicia agreed, and with the approval of the administrator my visit was scheduled for the following Monday.

I shall never forget that day. I met Alicia at her office, and she took me to the recreation area not far from the nurse's station, where a group of about twenty residents had been gathered for their morning exercise. As soon as we walked through the door, I was surrounded by men and women who seemed eager to gain my attention. They welcomed me with such warmth and acceptance that the tension I had been feeling since my arrival vanished in an instant. Some of the residents greeted me as though I was an old friend or a relative.

"Where have you been, dear?" asked Frieda as she took my hand and held it to her cheek in a gesture of affection.

"How is Freddie?" asked Marvin. "Is he here too?"

I didn't know who Freddie was, but I assured Marvin that Freddie would come to see him soon, and Marvin appeared to be pleased with my reply.

"I'm so glad you could come," exclaimed Agnes graciously. "This is going to be a wonderful party. All my friends are here."

Emily, who could no longer verbalize except in a sort of gibberish, linked her arm through mine and pulled me to a chair next to hers as Alicia and Mimi, her assistant, got everyone seated in a circle to begin the exercise session.

I was amazed at how attentive everyone was, and how well most of the residents were able to participate and follow the exercise routines Mimi called out and demonstrated, even those residents in wheelchairs.

After exercise, snacks and beverages were served. The rest of the morning passed quickly as the group was engaged in a variety of games. I noticed that several of the residents became restless and distracted after a short time. Some wandered off and paced down the hall, but most came back shortly to rejoin the group.

I learned a great deal about AD as the day progressed. I spent time on a one-on-one basis with as many residents as possible, seeking out some of the more passive ones as well as several who were in the last stages of the disease.

Some of the residents had retained excellent verbal skills and good memory recall to the point that it was difficult for me to notice any obvious signs of cognitive deterioration. Elizabeth, one of the most articulate residents, spoke to me about her job teaching English literature at a junior college. We got into a lively discussion about our favorite books and authors, including Edith Wharton, Henry James, and Charles Dickens. Elizabeth impressed me with her knowledge and her memory for detail. Just as I began to wonder what problems could possibly have caused her to live in an Alzheimer's facility, she said, "Well, it was a pleasure to talk to you. We must meet again soon, but I have to get ready to go to work now." And she got up and rushed down the hall to her room.

Later, when I mentioned the incident to the nursing supervisor, she explained that Elizabeth told the staff several times each day that she had to go to work.

"How do you handle that situation without upsetting her?" I asked.

"When she was first admitted here, we tried to convince her that she was retired," replied the nursing supervisor. "But she refused to accept that explanation and became very agitated and angry. Now we just tell her that it is a holiday or the weekend and the school is closed."

"Are you telling me you can use these explanations several times a day and she believes you?" I asked.

"Oh yes," replied the supervisor. "She doesn't remember from one moment to the next what she has been told. She has no short-term memory anymore. Anything we tell her is forgotten in five minutes or less. Her brain can no longer retain recent information."

I was truly astonished, considering that Elizabeth had such excellent recall of books, her job and other memories from her past.

In contrast to Elizabeth, some of the residents had great difficulties finding words to express themselves. However, that did not deter them from conversing with others.

Edward, a courtly gentleman of the old school, who was known to hold out a chair for a lady or give up his own seat to one, had a problem recalling words. He could start a conversation easily enough, but often had to pause midsentence to search his mind for a word he needed to complete it. If he came up empty, it was obviously upsetting to him. He would throw up his hands in defeat, shake his head, and let out a deep sigh, saying, "I am so sorry I can't find the word." If, as often happened, the person conversing with him discerned what he had meant to say and supplied the correct word, Edward repeated it several times and thanked the person. But by then he had usually forgotten what he had intended to say.

Antonia, on the other hand, was unconcerned about her verbal lapses. If she couldn't recall a word or, as happened frequently, lost her train of thought midsentence, she would let it trail off unfinished with the statement, "You know." And it was left up to you to figure out what she had meant to communicate. "You know" was an expression I would hear hundreds, if not thousands of times during the next eight years of working with Alzheimer's patients.

Then there was Emily, who could only babble, yet that babbling along with her smile and her gestures, communicated very effectively. In the afternoon, she approached me, as she had in the morning, and took my arm to walk me through the enclosed garden. This garden, adjacent to the dayroom, was accessible to the residents from sunup to sundown, weather permitting.

Emily walked me along the garden path babbling continuously. "Come on, we need some exercise and I would like your companionship. Isn't this a pretty place? Look at the flowers, aren't they lovely? Let's sit down on this bench for a while. I really like you. I'm glad you like me too. Thank you for coming with me." All of this Emily communicated to me. I had no idea whether she understood any of the words I said to her, but it was evident that she enjoyed our conversation, and so did I.

It amazed me that even some of the most seriously impaired residents responded to my visits with a certain degree of attentiveness, if only for a moment.

Olga, aged ninety-two, whose hands were so contracted that her fingers were bent into her palms, smiled in response to my greeting. That brief smile was all she could manage, according to the staff. Olga had end-stage AD, and she could no longer move any part of her body.

That first day at Magnolia Manor passed very quickly, but within the first two hours of meeting the residents I knew I wanted to work with them. I could not even imagine walking away and never seeing them again.

My head was filled with my impressions of the residents, the staff and the facility, all of which were positive. And I was fascinated by what I had so far learned of this complex disease. At the same time, I recognized what a challenge it would be to meet the individual as well as the collective needs of this varied population in providing appropriate and therapeutic recreational activities. I was deeply cognizant of how much I had yet to learn about Alzheimer's disease.

At the end of that Monday, I formally accepted the position. As I filled out the documents for my personnel file, Alicia confessed, "I have been holding my breath all day, hoping you would take the job. I could tell by the residents' reaction to you that they really liked you and felt comfortable with you. I told you you'd be a natural." She then proceeded to familiarize me with the specifics of my job.

I was to work Saturdays and Sundays from nine to five. Nursing assistants would be available to help gather the residents for the activity programs, and one of them would be assigned to assist with serving snacks, but I would be the only person working in the recreation department on those days. I was given what I considered a somewhat superficial briefing regarding my duties, and it was left up to me to structure the program. "After all, you have so many years of experience working in recreation, this will be a snap for you," reasoned Alicia.

I cannot say that I shared her confidence in my abilities. I could see that Alzheimer's patients needed a very different kind of program than what was appropriate for psychiatric patients. When I asked for a schedule of past weekend programs, I was informed that the facility had not had any weekend coverage for some time. Prior to that, there had been some volunteers who had come in for a few hours on weekends.

Alicia had one more surprise for me. She asked me to conduct a religious service on Sunday mornings.

"Most of our residents have been accustomed to going to church on Sunday. That's primarily what our volunteer did on Sundays, she conducted a service. It meant a lot to the residents and they enjoyed it immensely," Alicia explained.

I was dumbfounded. I had been baptized and confirmed in the Lutheran church, and attended church services regularly as a child, but I had not belonged to any organized religious group in many years.

Alicia, noting my obvious discomfort, said, "Look, it's no big deal. Just say a few prayers, read a short passage from the Bible. The most important part of the whole service for the resident is singing the hymns."

"I don't sing very well, and I only know a few hymns," I stammered.

"Don't worry about that," said Alicia soothingly. "Most of our residents can sing them. They may not remember what they had for breakfast, or where they are, but they do know their hymns—and they love to sing. Besides, we have Bessie who will play the piano. She used to be the organist in her church. She knows all the hymns."

I was only mildly reassured. But wanting to work at Magnolia Manor as much as I did, I assured Alicia that I would do my best.

I had less than a week, four days to be exact, to plan my weekend program of recreational activities. I hoped that during that time I could gain enough knowledge about AD to feel more confident about my job.

I went to the public library and found several books that dealt with AD. The one that looked most promising was called *The 36-Hour Day: A Family Guide to Caring for Persons with Alzheimer's Disease, Related Dementing Illnesses, and Memory Loss in Later Life.*[1] It had originally been published in 1981, but this second edition was published in 1991. As I browsed through it, I saw that it covered a wide range of topics but gave scant information about AD patients in long-term care settings and about the day-to-day activities most suitable for them. Then I noticed in the appendix that there was something called The Alzheimer's Association, which had chapters throughout the United States.

I placed a call to the local chapter. When I told the lady who answered the phone about my job at Magnolia Manor, she was impressed. "Congratulations," she said, "Magnolia Manor is one of the very best facilities for Alzheimer's patients in the entire state." I was very pleased that I had, through sheer luck, gotten a job at such a superior facility.

My phone call to the Alzheimer's Association proved to be another piece of good luck, as well as good timing. I was informed that on Thursday and Friday of this week, a seminar for caregivers was scheduled at a local hotel. The seminar, "Creative Intervention with the Alzheimer's Patient," was conducted by Mary Lucero, a licensed nursing-home administrator. I was to learn that Ms. Lucero was a woman of many accomplishments. *She is the founder and president of Geriatric Resources, Inc., a company that has developed a series of sensory stimulation products for Alzheimer's patients. In 1989 she was a recipient of a Small Business Innovation Research grant from the National Institute of Aging (NIA) and has also testified before the U.S. Senate Select Committee on Aging. Her testimony focused on the 1990 enactment of the Nursing Home Reform Law, OBRA (Omnibus Budget Reconciliation Act of 1987) and its impact on Alzheimer's Care.*[2]

The seminar seemed tailor-made for my needs, and I could not have had a better teacher. The lectures were informative, illuminating, and inspiring. Ever since, I have thought of Mary Lucero as my mentor, though we have never spoken personally. The videotapes of her lectures continue to be the best source of information on caregiving methods for Alzheimer's patients in long-term care settings.

Thanks to Mary Lucero, I started my job at Magnolia Manor with a solid base of knowledge about Alzheimer's disease and effective caregiving strategies. Most importantly, I came equipped with lots of creative ideas to incorporate into my weekend programs. In the ensuing years, I never missed a seminar given by Mary Lucero if it was held in a location accessible to me. Throughout the years of my work with Alzheimer's patients, she has been my inspiration. I only wish that every caregiver who works with such patients in the nursing homes could be so fortunate.

1. Nancy L. Mace, MA, Peter V. Rabins, MD, MPH. *The 36-Hour Day: A Family Guide to Caring for Persons with Alzheimer's Disease, Related Dementing Illnesses, and Memory Loss in Later Life*, (Baltimore: Johns Hopkins University Press, 1991).
2. ibid.
3. Reported by the *Small Business Development Center News and Program Update*, College of Business Administration, University of Central Florida, September-December 1991.

I'm Richard. Everybody knows me.

—Richard

Chapter 4

When I arrived at Magnolia Manor early on Saturday morning for the first day of work, I was still preoccupied with all that I had learned that week. I had not had much time to work out a detailed schedule of activities, although I had a general plan in mind. I knew I wanted to include a Cognitive Stimulation Program, but I had decided to begin the day with exercise, the same exercise program that was conducted each weekday morning.

The CNAs had already gathered the residents in a circle in the dayroom. I was greeted with the same warmth the residents had exhibited the first time we had met.

I more or less followed the same routines and movements I'd seen Alicia use but added some livelier music to my program. I had found several appropriate musical tapes in the recreation room cupboard, one featuring Herb Alpers and his band.

The first hour passed quickly. When it was time for midmorning snacks, the two CNAs assisting me seated the residents at the tables while I went into the tiny auxiliary kitchen adjacent to the dayroom to get the coffee.

I was in the midst of setting up a tray with cream, sugar, cups, and spoons, when I heard a splashing sound behind me. I turned around and saw a male resident, one I had not met before, with his pants around his ankles, urinating into the tall metal garbage can that stood against the wall. I was utterly astonished. No one had prepared me for such a situation.

"What are you doing?" I said, realizing what a stupid question that was as soon as the words were out of my mouth.

The man just grinned at me and said, "Hi," as if what he was doing was the most natural thing in the world. He did not appear to be the least bit embarrassed, while I could feel myself turning red from my neck to the top of my head.

When he was finished, the man said, "Bye," and proceeded to shuffle out of the room, his pants still bunched around his ankles.

"Wait a minute," I said, "You forgot to pull up your pants."

He paused, looked down at himself, but appeared to be at a loss as to what to do. "What's your name?" I asked, as I moved cautiously a little closer to him.

"I'm Richard," he replied. "Everybody knows me," and he flashed me another cheerful grin.

"I'm glad to know you, Richard," I said, and introduced myself. I pointed to his pants and asked, "May I help you with your clothes, Richard?"

He nodded his head and I moved in to pull up his pants while I invited him to join us for snacks. Richard said, "Hi," again and held out his hand to me. I shook it with my right while I zipped up his fly with my left hand. Then I took him to the dayroom where the snacks had just arrived. I returned to the kitchen, washed my hands vigorously, grabbed the tray, and rejoined the group in the dayroom.

Later, when I had a chance to talk about the incident with Diane, one of the nurses, she laughed. "Did he do that again? I'm sorry nobody warned you."

"You mean he has done this before?" I asked.

"Oh yes," replied Diane, "He does that every chance he gets, and not just in the kitchen can. Any can or wastebasket will do, wherever he can find one."

"I had to pull up his pants. He didn't seem to know how to do that, yet he introduced himself appropriately," I told Diane.

She laughed again, "Did he say 'I'm Richard. Everybody knows me'?"

"Yes," I replied. "He said it exactly like that."

"And did he say 'Hi' and 'Bye'?" asked Diane.

"Yes, he said that too," I confirmed.

"Then he used all the words he can still say," Diane told me.

She paused, looking pensive; after a moment she continued, "Please, understand that I did not mean to make fun of Richard when I laughed just now. I mean, what he does is funny, but what happened to him and to all of our residents is heartbreaking. Sometimes we have to laugh at the behaviors we see here every day. If we thought only of the disease that has caused them, it would be impossible to come to work here every day."

I assured Diane that I understood and appreciated what she told me, knowing how important it is to maintain a sense of humor when working in an environment where one is constantly reminded of the tragedies of life.

Diane reached behind her to the shelf where the residents' medical charts were kept and pulled one out.

"Here," she said, as she handed it to me. "This is Richard's chart. It may be interesting for you to read it."

I sat down behind the nurses' station and began to read.

Richard was born and raised in a small town near Miami, Florida. He was the oldest of three siblings. His father died when Richard was seven years old. His mother went to work as a maid for a wealthy family in the area. At age fourteen, Richard dropped out of school to take a job as a gardener's assistant for the same family. At age eighteen, he enlisted in the U.S. Army and was shipped to Europe where he participated in the invasion of Italy.

Upon his return to the United States at the end of WWII, he completed high school, and then went to college on the GI Bill. He majored in physics and chemistry, and taught high school thereafter for several years, while he continued his education. He married Ruth M. in 1953, and they raised four children together. After Richard received his PhD in chemistry at the University of

Florida, the family moved to Massachusetts, where he had obtained a teaching position at a prestigious university. In 1983 he retired and moved with his wife and their youngest daughter back to Florida. His wife died of cancer in 1985.

It was around that time, according to his daughter, that Richard began to exhibit episodes of confusion and forgetfulness. Initially these symptoms were attributed to his grief over the loss of his wife, and he was treated with antidepressant medication. However, over time his condition deteriorated further, and in 1988 he was diagnosed with AD. Shortly thereafter, Richard was admitted to Magnolia Manor. His daughter Althea visits him frequently and continues to be involved in his care.

After snack time was over, I invited Richard to join us for the rest of the morning's program. At first, he did sit down to watch his peers but refused to participate. Within less than five minutes, he became restless and wandered off, pacing the hallways.

In the afternoon, we played a series of cognitive stimulation games. I had made up a set of flash cards of simple words the night before. As I held these aloft, one at a time, several residents read the word aloud and I then asked them to name the opposite word. I also had a variety of objects on hand for those residents who were unable to read and asked them to identify the objects. At this point I wanted to get to know the residents and their level of cognitive abilities—their interests and their ability to maintain focused attention, their ability to process information.

Over the following weeks, I developed a whole series of cognitive and sensory stimulation games and collected props that were helpful in triggering memories. But on this first day, I managed with flash cards, music, and what props I could find on the premises. After afternoon snacks, we had a sing-along.

Again, I had approached Richard to join us, but he declined and resumed his pacing. When I asked Diane if he ever attended any of the recreation programs, she shook her head.

"As far as I know he has never attended anything. He is very restless—always has been—since he came here. He spends most of his time pacing. We have all tried to encourage him, but he just doesn't seem able to settle down. Sometimes he wears himself out to the point of exhaustion.

"We have asked his daughter's permission to get him onto a tranquilizer to slow him down, but she decided she would rather see him pace than take the risk of his becoming a 'passive vegetable,' as she put it."

At the end of the day I was exhausted, but also elated. I felt that my first day with the residents had gone well. They had obviously enjoyed the program and had, for the most part, been more attentive than I had anticipated. The CNAs had been a big help, and I also appreciated the positive feedback I received from the nurses.

In spite of the good feelings my first day at Magnolia Manor had engendered, it was with some trepidation that I entered the facility on Sunday morning. After all, I had never before been called upon to conduct a religious service, and I felt I was on shaky ground.

I had spent most of the previous evening preparing for this event with the help of a Bible, a prayer book, and a list of the residents' favorite hymns, which Alicia had given me.

At first, I had found it daunting to come up with a program that would be appropriate and meaningful to a group of people with limited attention spans and at such varied stages of cognitive impairments. I knew that many of the residents found it difficult to sit still for any length of time, and I had visions of them getting up in the midst of the service and walking away.

Eventually I realized that these thoughts were entirely unproductive. I changed my approach and posed myself the following question: What did I want the residents to get out of this service? The answer came quickly: I hoped they would experience a measure of comfort and joy. "Yes," I thought, "I want them to have, above all, a joyful experience."

I knew they loved to sing, and according to the nurses, many also recalled prayers and Bible verses that they had learned in childhood. Accordingly, my formula was to keep it simple, use familiar prayers, recite one or two uplifting passages of Scripture, and have them sing lots of hymns in between.

Once I had selected the prayers and the readings for the service, I turned my attention to what I should wear. I felt it should be something festive but also bright and cheerful. Something that I hoped would keep the residents' attention focused on me during the service, thus minimizing distraction.

In the back of my closet I found a Mexican dress of white cotton, embroidered all over with large cross-stitched flowers in a brilliant array of colors. It had looked great in Mexico where it blended in with the many colorful garments worn by the native population, but back in New York it had always seemed too gaudy to me, and I had not worn it in years. Now it seemed to be the perfect garment for my purpose.

So, wearing my colorful Mexican dress, I was as ready as I ever would be to lead the Sunday morning service. The furniture in the spacious dayroom had been pushed back against the walls, and the CNAs had set up six rows of folding chairs, leaving space to accommodate the wheelchair bound.

I opened the lid of the piano and arranged the sheet music for the hymns in proper sequence on the stand. Bessie, who was to play the piano, had not yet arrived, but I was assured by the staff that she was getting ready to join us.

Several of the residents were already seated, and the CNAs were bringing in more of them. I plugged in the cassette player and put in a cassette of Bach's sacred music. It sounded wonderful, just like in a church, thanks to the excellent acoustics of this large room.

I helped the CNAs bring in and seat the rest of the residents. Soon every seat and every space was filled, and we had to add additional chairs for the latecomers.

I was impressed. The residents sat silently, patiently, expectantly, listening to the music as if they were actually in a church. After they had all been seated, I turned off the tape and wished everyone a cheerful "Good Morning," which they returned in unison.

Then I gave the invocation: "This is the day the Lord has made . . ." After which I signaled to Bessie, who began to play our first hymn, "Amazing Grace." Aside from playing the piano well, Bessie also had a beautiful soprano voice. I was grateful for that, as my own voice was rather scratchy.

Most of the residents joined in the singing, and there were several other good voices, including the baritone of seventy-nine-year-old Lloyd, who was wheelchair bound, having lost one of his legs to diabetes. Several of the residents who could no longer use language or did not remember the words hummed along.

We sang a second hymn, "What a Friend We Have in Jesus." Then I recited the Twenty-Third Psalm. I noted that an impressive number of residents knew every word and recited it with me.

We had just finished, and I was about to announce the name of the next hymn, when Marvin left his seat and began to push his way out of his row amidst loud protests from those seated there.

"Marvin, please sit down, we are going to sing again," I called out to him, but he ignored me. He walked up front, holding both arms aloft and shouting, "My turn, my turn!" He stopped about three feet to my left, faced the "congregation" and proceeded to give a speech.

"Ladies and gentlemen, thank you for coming. This is a very special occasion and we must celebrate. I'm sorry my wife can't be here. She would if she could, but she couldn't and she wouldn't . . ."

By now, the residents had become restless and angry. Chairs scraped, murmurs and growls of disapproval filled the room. Ethel shouted, "Shut up, shut up, you snake!" She waved her arms wildly toward Marvin. Someone else yelled, "You are in the house of the Lord, and He will smite you with a vengeance if you don't stop babbling."

Tiny eighty-one-year-old Vardell curled herself up into a ball (thank God, she had been seated in a club chair). She covered her ears and started to whimper. Hanna, who was seated next to her, let out a bloodcurdling howl.

It was bedlam—and I had lost control. It had all happened so fast. In an instant, my worshipful, well-behaved congregation had fallen apart. My worst nightmare had come to pass. But before I could even think about what to do, several CNAs and nurses came to the rescue. One escorted Marvin away from the group (he was still talking about his wife who wouldn't and couldn't), and the others fanned out to calm and reassure those who were most upset. Vardell, who couldn't stop crying, was taken out.

I managed to reassure Ethel and several others that we would continue the service as soon as order was restored. I noticed that holding their hands for a moment and smiling at them went a long way toward getting them to sit down and remain calm.

As soon as it was quiet I announced the next hymn and directed Bessie to start playing. She played a few bars of "How Great Thou Art," then stopped, looking confused as the voices of the congregation died down. I walked over to her and pointed to the sheet music. "Bessie," I said, "Go ahead and start again." I even hummed the first few bars to reorient her. But Bessie didn't seem to hear me. She just sat immobile, staring into space.

Meanwhile several of the residents had gotten restless again. I could see them squirming in their seats. Two got up and left. I tried again to get Bessie to respond to my request. Suddenly she snapped her fingers and began to play. But it wasn't the hymn she had been asked to play. It was a boogie-woogie tune.

In an instant, the congregation came alive; they were transformed. They clapped their hands and stamped their feet to the beat of the music. They swayed and hummed along with it. Where a moment before they had been angry at Marvin, they now looked positively cheerful and happy.

I decided to go with the flow. Who's to say boogie-woogie is inappropriate during a religious service? Not I. After all, my goal had been to make the service a joyful event for the residents, and Bessie had found a way to make it so, better than I could have done.

But I did want to give the Lord his due. So after Bessie finished playing, I said, "That was wonderful, Bessie. Thank you very much," and clapped my hands to applaud her. The group followed suit to show their appreciation.

I turned to the congregation, held my prayer book aloft and announced, "Let us pray." Everyone quieted down and most bowed their heads. I recited the prayer I had selected because I felt it would be particularly uplifting and comforting to those who are afflicted with Alzheimer's.

> *Oh God, let us move into each new day with courage, knowing you are by our side, when hope and good cheer fail to carry us through. When confronted by mystery, help us to remember that we do not have to know everything. May we rest our hearts in Thee, at least for today. This we pray and also, as You taught us . . .*

Then I recited the Lord's Prayer, and everyone who still remembered it and could use language joined in. We sang one more hymn; I gave the Benediction, and the service was over.

Once more, I played the Bach cassette, and we took the residents to the dining room for lunch, the glorious music soaring around us.

Of the approximately 1.5 million nursing home residents in the
United States, one fifth suffer from symptoms of depression.
Up to 40 percent of residents with dementia have both behavioral
and psychiatric symptoms.
—The American Association for Geriatric Psychiatry[1]

Chapter 5

Although I enjoyed working with the residents at Magnolia Manor, my income from this part-time job, combined with my earnings from a second part-time job in retail, were not sufficient to cover my living expenses, and I continued to search for full-time employment.

Within less than three months, I obtained a position that would be both challenging and rewarding. A community mental health agency in a nearby county was initiating a new program to provide mental health services, on site, to eligible residents of long-term care facilities, such as nursing homes. This service had just recently been introduced in the state of Florida and was funded by Medicaid. I was hired as coordinator of the program in the county adjacent to the one where I then lived.

It had long been recognized by gerontologists and other health-care professionals serving the elderly that when mental health issues are not conscientiously addressed, there is a much more rapid decline in the general health and functioning of the individual. Yet according to the American Association of Geriatric Psychiatry, the majority of the nation's nursing homes have failed to provide adequate mental health services for those residents who suffer from mental illness.

The state of Florida, which has for decades been home for the largest population of senior citizens per capita in the United States, has always been in the forefront of improving services for their seniors. Therefore, it was not surprising that this state took the lead in initiating a mental health service for its nursing home residents.

The primary goal of the Mental Health Nursing Home Program (MHNH) was to improve the quality of life for those residents who exhibited impaired function due to mental illness and residents who are cognitively impaired due to Alzheimer's disease and other forms of dementia. The services provided included individual and group therapy, crisis intervention, consultation, as needed, with caregivers, support services for family members, and participation in the nursing homes' interdisciplinary care-plan creations and reviews.

The nursing homes that chose to participate in the program (it was not mandatory and several declined) signed a contract with their community mental health agency. Counselors designated "nursing home specialists" were assigned to each of the facilities to implement the program. Eligibility and need for services were determined through an extensive assessment process. In addition, a resident's inclusion in the program had to be agreed to by the resident or the resident's health-care surrogate and approved by the resident's attending physician. Those residents who required medication for their mental condition were regularly visited by the psychiatrist who prescribed it.

Since the program was an entirely new concept of services, there was no one who could tell us, based on experience, what it would be like to provide mental health services within the nursing home setting. We were breaking new ground and establishing protocols along the way.

The majority of the nursing home residents who became MHNH clients had dementia, primarily of the Alzheimer's type, and many were depressed and/or exhibited serious behavior problems.

The staff we hired for the program all had experience working with the mentally ill in a variety of settings, but none of them had ever worked in a nursing home or with Alzheimer's patients. Although my own experience with them had been of short duration, I had been fortunate that it had been gained at Magnolia Manor, a state-of-the-art facility that provided outstanding care for its residents. I had learned a great deal there about AD in a very short time.

One of my first duties, before we even set foot into the nursing homes, was to do an in-service on Alzheimer's disease for our newly created nursing home specialists who were as enthusiastic and excited as I was about participating in this new program.

As to the practical aspects of working in the nursing homes, they were a real challenge, especially in the beginning. We had to be mindful, at all times, not to interfere with the established routines of the facilities. Providing services for our clients demanded much flexibility and juggling of schedules.

Although we had been assured by the management of each facility, that they were pleased to have our services, only one of them made an effort to provide us with a working space where we could bring our clients for individual counseling sessions and where my staff and I could meet in privacy to discuss confidential issues, as needed. This facility cleaned out a large storage closet for us and put in a desk and two chairs. In the other nursing homes, we had no such private space.

Individual counseling sessions took place in the residents' room, whenever possible. However, since most residents had a roommate, we often had to wait for this person to leave the room so we could have the privacy we needed. It was not unusual for us to conduct individual sessions out-of-doors, in a secluded area of the patio, or even while taking the resident for a walk.

Fortunately, most of our clients were delighted to be taken out for their counseling sessions. For some of them it was a rare treat to be out-of-doors.

For group therapy, we met with our clients in the dining rooms. Scheduling these sessions also required flexibility on our part as the dining rooms were off-limits to us for extended periods each day while the room was being cleared after breakfast, while tables were being set for the midday meal, and until after the midday meal cleanup.

In most facilities, the dining room was also utilized for religious services, for entertainment, and in some facilities even for exercise and recreation programs.

Since privacy was not an issue with the cognitive and sensory stimulation programs we initiated for the Alzheimer's residents, we were able to conduct these sessions in one of the dayrooms were nonparticipants were usually present.

As program coordinator, my workday was divided between administrative duties, supervision of staff, and providing clinical services for my clients, who were located in several different facilities. Approximately 40 percent of my workday was devoted to client services. This was by far my favorite part of the job, and I envied my staff who were able to spend the majority of their workday with clients, although they too had to devote time to paperwork.

A typical workday for me started at 8:30 AM at one of the facilities where I attended to some of the never-ending mountain of paperwork, met briefly with my staff and/or with nursing-home personnel to discuss any issues that required my attention. But I always looked forward to leading the group sessions for the Alzheimer's residents at several of the nursing homes we served.

Cognitive and sensory stimulation group session for the Alzheimer's residents were scheduled daily at all of the facilities served by the MHNH program. Since the cognitive and language skills of the participants varied from mild to severe impairments, we presented short segments of very simple to incrementally more complex mental exercises, such as word games, sentence completion, arithmetic, object identification, and reminiscing. We used flash cards and a variety of props that helped to jog memories and to stimulate the mind and senses. We also employed music and physical exercises daily to keep everyone alert. Sing-alongs and ball-tossing exercises were the group's favorite activities.

In addition to promoting alertness, mental stimulation, and a sense of accomplishment, we encouraged social interaction between group members. Everyone, no matter how seriously impaired, became more animated and cheerful during our sessions. Over time, we added other activities to the program. But in every session, humor, fun, and laughter played a large role, and the residents loved them.

After group I usually saw several of my clients in individual sessions, then moved on to another facility to touch base with my staff there and to see clients who were scheduled for a session that day. By four or four-thirty in the afternoon I usually headed back to our home office at the mental health agency, where I might meet with my supervisor, the director of the MHNH program, and/or attend to other administrative duties.

Often, before calling it a day I returned to one of the facilities to see a client who had been having a difficult day and could gain from a little extra attention, I rarely headed home much before six-thirty or even seven o'clock. Sometimes I returned after dinner, to spend time with a depressed client, especially if that person no longer had any family who might have provided some emotional support. It should be noted that such visits were not billable to Medicaid, nor did any of us in the program ever ask for or receive compensation for any overtime we worked.

In addition, there were many other details to attend to in a workday such as meetings with clients' family members, attending care-plan meetings, assisting nursing home staff in crisis resolutions, weekly meetings with staff, and always the paperwork—including writing program evaluation reports, quarterly job-performance evaluations of mental health nursing home specialists, as well as writing progress reports in the medical carts of each of my clients.

There were many challenges to meet, and there never seemed to be enough time to do all that needed to be done. Fortunately, the facilities we served were all located within a short distance from each other and from our home office, so it took only a few minutes to drive from one to the other.

In spite of all the obstacles we encountered in our work in the nursing homes, we loved our work with the residents. And it was evident from the responsiveness of our clients and the feedback we received from them, from their families and even from some of the nursing home caregivers, that the mental health program added a much-needed and valuable component to nursing home care.

---

1. Kate McDuffie, American Association of Geriatric Psychiatry: Quote from a report on Mental Health Treatment for Nursing Home Residents by an Interdisciplinary Panel of Geriatric Experts led by the American Association of Geriatric Psychiatry and The American Association of Psychiatry. http://www.aagp online.org/news/pressreleases.asp, Sept. 2, 2003.

I can go any place I want, and you can't stop me.
—Sophie

Chapter 6

Sophie had been famous in her community for her exquisite garden. Year after year, she won prizes for her outstanding fruits and vegetables, and for the beauty of her flowers. Throughout the planting season, Sophie was up and working in her garden before sunrise. She also enjoyed taking long walks through the fields and along the roads of her native Maine. She knew the names of most of the plants, trees, and wildflowers that grew in the area. According to her son, Michael, Sophie spent most of her life out-of-doors. "Even a blizzard couldn't keep her in the house."

She greeted the first snow of the season with the exuberance and delight of a child. At age sixty-eight, she thought nothing of trudging up a steep hill with her grandchildren and whizzing down, at breakneck speed, seated on a sled behind a child.

She was enchanted by the glittering stars in the night sky, and taught her children the names of the constellations in the solar system when they were barely old enough to talk. She also taught them reverence for nature.

"My mother was totally in tune with the rhythm of the natural world," commented Michael. "She used to say, 'Children, we are still living in the Garden of Eden, only most people don't know it.'"

Sophie is seventy-nine years old now. She has Alzheimer's

disease and has been living at the nursing home for the past three months. She is severely cognitively impaired. She is in reasonably good physical health, but is emotionally fragile. She is still adjusting to the drastic change in her environment. What appears to be most difficult for her to accept, as it is for most newcomers to the nursing home, is to be physically confined to the facility.

Sophie's children and grandchildren visit her regularly and take her out for short walks in the garden. They also bring her potted plants, hoping to reawaken her interest in growing things, but this has not been successful. Sophie no longer appears to make the connection between the nurturing of plants and their growth. The staff tries to remember to water her plants for her, but they often forget, or are too busy to take the time, and eventually the plants whither and die.

However, Sophie is attracted by the flowers in the facility's garden, which she can see through the windows. This view seems to trigger her desire to be out-of-doors. Except when she is occupied with purposeful activities, such as eating meals or attending recreation programs, Sophie paces from exit door to exit door, rattling, hitting, and kicking these doors in an effort to escape.

Only the sustained attention of staff can interrupt this behavior. Unfortunately, staff are unable to devote the majority of their time to one resident on a continuous basis. Often Sophie's frustration at her inability to open a door will escalate into a full-blown catastrophic outburst, especially when staff tell her to stop her behavior and to get away from the door.

One morning, after the conclusion of my cognitive and sensory stimulation group, I was on my way to the activity room to store the props I had been using, when I observed the following scene taking place at the other end of the hall.

The medication nurse was standing at her cart, near one of the exit doors, when Sophie walked past her and began to rattle the door. Unfortunately, someone had failed to secure the lock, and the door flew open.

Just as Sophie stepped across the threshold, the nurse whipped around, tackled her, and pulled her back inside, shouting at her, "You know you are not allowed to go out that door!"

Sophie was so startled that she literally jumped as she screamed, "I can go any place I want, and you can't stop me!"

The nurse continued to berate her as she locked the door. "Sophie, you know very well that I can't let you go out there by yourself. Why don't you behave yourself and go to the recreation program? Go on." She waved her hand for emphasis in the direction of the dayroom.

Sophie was enraged. She took two steps back, then ran at the nurse, pushed her up against the wall, and kicked and pummeled her with her fists, screaming, "Bitch, I hate you! I'm going to kill you."

The entire incident happened in less than a minute, by which time I had traveled the distance between us. As I reached them, both Sophie and the nurse stood frozen and trembling, glaring at each other. I took advantage of this moment of suspended animation to divert Sophie's attention away from the nurse. I called out, "Good morning, Sophie!"

Sophie turned around instantly. The scowl on her face dissolved into a smile as she registered my presence then reached out for the vase of flowers I held out to her, one of the props I had used that morning.

"Ah, what a beautiful bouquet," she exclaimed, "Are these for me?"

"Yes," I told her, and suggested that we take the flowers to her room.

Without a backward glance, Sophie accompanied me to her room, reminiscing gaily about the variety of flowers she used to grow in her garden.

The crisis was over. Sophie had already forgotten that just moments before, she had been assaulting the nurse.

Meanwhile, several staff members had come to the assistance of the nurse who had sustained several painful bruises and was badly shaken.

As I took Sophie away from the site of the incident, I wondered if the medication nurse understood that it was she, not Sophie, who had precipitated the crisis that caused this resident to assault her.

During the years I have worked in the nursing homes, I have witnessed many such incidents in which caregivers provoked a resident in such a manner that a minor problem quickly escalated into a crisis situation that resulted in a catastrophic outburst and assault upon the caregiver.

In one of her lectures, Mary Lucero[1] stated that 90 percent of catastrophic outbursts by Alzheimer's residents are due to inappropriate approaches by caregivers and/or a nursing home environment that has not been adapted to the special needs of the Alzheimer's residents.

In this instance the nurse used poor judgment in her interaction with Sophie. Her behavior was confrontational, disrespectful and demeaning to this resident.

Sophie's quest to elope continued unabated. On several occasions, she actually succeeded in getting out of the building. At least twice, she duped a visitor into escorting her to the front door (which was unlocked), convincing each person that she was also a visitor who had simply lost her way. Although Sophie was confused and cognitively impaired, she had retained good language and social skills. She continued to be well-groomed, always carried her handbag, and wore a pair of black dress shoes with one-and-a-half-inch heels, unlike most residents who preferred to wear slippers or low-heeled, comfortable shoes.

On casual acquaintance it was not apparent that Sophie was in any way impaired. Her admission that she could not find the exit from the facility was not a reason to question her status. Many first-time visitors had difficulty finding their way out of the building and had to ask someone for directions.

In none of her escape attempts did Sophie get far. She could usually be found on the grounds of the facility, most often in the section that was planted with flowers. The difficulty arose in getting her to come back into the building. She rarely agreed to come willingly, and there were times when she fought like a wildcat, heaping verbal and physical abuse on the staff who had been assigned to bring her back.

One morning as I drove into the facility's parking lot, I noticed a group of staff members crowded together on the lawn. They were moving about, and there was much shouting. Obviously, there was some sort of crisis in progress. I quickly parked my car and ran over to assist with whatever the problem was.

As I got closer, I saw that it was Sophie who had been surrounded on all sides. She was swinging her handbag at the staff, kicking and shouting obscenities. She was in a towering rage, slippery as an eel, shaking herself free from the hands that were trying to restrain her.

I was appalled at the behavior of the staff. They were obviously ignorant of the most basic rules of crisis intervention. And I wondered who had made the ill-conceived decision to send a posse out after one lone resident.

I broke through the middle of the group and yelled as loud as I could, "Leave Sophie alone! Step back, all of you!" The staff was so startled that they obeyed and stepped back a few paces, but they continued to surround Sophie. I motioned with my arms, "All of you, please go away! Leave me alone with Sophie." Again the staff retreated a few steps, but I could sense their hostility toward me. Several of them made disparaging remarks. "Who the hell does she think she is?"

I was well aware that they were shocked and offended by my rudeness. But for the moment I had to ignore that. I would apologize to them later.

But at this moment I was focused on rescuing Sophie from herself, as well as from the staff.

I motioned to the staff to get completely out of sight, which they did. I then turned to Sophie who had been standing still, watching my interaction with them. I smiled and said, "Hi, Sophie, I'm going for a walk. Would you like to join me?"

"Sure," she said, and I could hear the relief in the tone of her voice. "You know I love to walk. I'm glad you made all those bad people go away, they wanted to hurt me."

"Oh no, Sophie. They didn't mean any harm. They were concerned that you might get lost out here, all by yourself," I explained.

"I was so scared," continued Sophie. "I don't like it when people grab at me."

"I know, that didn't feel comfortable, but it's over now," I said, and then changed the subject, hoping she would forget the entire unpleasant incident as quickly as possible.

The grounds of this facility were exceptionally large and beautifully landscaped. One of its most attractive features was a pond on which a family of ducks had made their home.

We walked around the pond at a leisurely pace. Sophie was reveling in being out-of-doors on a beautiful day. She took deep appreciative breaths. "Oh, what wonderful fresh air," she cried. She pointed to a clump of daisies at the edge of the path. "Aren't these flowers just lovely? You know," she reminisced, "I used to pick armloads of wildflowers in the meadows near our home and arrange them into bouquets for every room in the house. My husband used to say, 'Sophie, no one can transform a room the way you do with your flowers. Oh, I'm a lucky man to have you for a wife.'"

I think Sophie could happily have walked all day. But it was getting very hot and humid and we both needed to go inside. I said, "Sophie, we need to get out of the sun now. I think we should go in."

"I'm fine," she replied. "I love being in the sun."

I suggested, "We could go to the dining room for a midmorning snack."

"No, I don't think so," said Sophie. "We can do that later."

A few minutes later, I tried again. "Sophie, you know it's almost time for lunch. We really should go in or you'll miss it."

"I'm not going to eat lunch today. I'm not hungry," Sophie declared and bent down to pull some weeds from a flower bed.

I spent another five minutes wracking my brain to come up with something that would convince Sophie to come inside.

"Sophie, you know your daughter may be on her way to visit with you. I'm sure you wouldn't want to miss her." There, that should do it, I thought

But Sophie didn't take the bait. "Susan can find me right here if she wants me," she said, and continued to pull up stray weeds.

I was running out of ideas. We had been out here for almost an hour, and I had several other clients I needed to see. Finally I said, "Sophie, I'm so thirsty. I think I'm going to faint if I don't get a drink soon."

Sophie looked at me sharply, "Honey, why didn't you say so before? I do declare you look downright puny." With that, she straightened up, tossed away the weeds, linked her arm through mine, and pulled me toward the front door of the facility.

"You know," she said as we came into the lobby, "I've never been here before, but it looks like a nice place."

I walked her to the dining room where a sing-along was in progress, and she joined the group. She had already forgotten her desire to stay out in the garden.

Later that day I met with the staff and apologized that I had been rude to them. But I also explained the reason for my behavior and took the opportunity to tell them why their confrontation with Sophie had frightened her and triggered a panic reaction.

"When I first arrived at the scene I could tell that Sophie was terrified. She was beyond cooperating with you, and you would have had to bring her back into the building by force. So I had to play good cop, bad cop, to get you to back off, to give Sophie time to calm down and to gain her trust."

My apologies were only grudgingly accepted. It took several weeks and much effort on my part to regain the staff's goodwill toward me. But I had no regrets. I had done what I considered necessary to rescue Sophie from a traumatizing experience.

In their attempt to bring Sophie back into the building, the staff had violated several of the most basic rules of crisis intervention.

In their *Nonviolent Crisis Intervention*® training program, the Crisis Prevention Institute, Inc. (CPI) teaches the following approaches, which are paraphrased and summarized here for length and applicability:[2]

1. The crisis team must assess the individual's behavior and must decide how much staff is needed to defuse the crisis.

Sophie's escape from the facility could, initially, hardly have been classified as a crisis.

She was still on the grounds of the facility and was not in any immediate danger, nor was she a danger to anyone else. There was no need for five or six people to come to her rescue. One staff person, using a nonthreatening friendly approach, could have gotten Sophie back into the building, without incident.

2. Only one person should approach the individual. In cases where there is a crisis team, the team leader, or the person who knows the individual best, should be the one to intervene.

Instead, the staff surrounded Sophie as a group, thus triggering in her feelings of fear and powerlessness as she perceived herself to be trapped.

3. Do not encroach personal space. As a rule allow at least three feet distance between yourself and the individual. Proximity can be perceived as a threat.

The staff had grossly violated this rule by getting right into Sophie's face, hardly giving her space to breathe.

4. Verbal communication should be supportive to the individual. Paraverbal communication, which consists of tone, volume and cadence of voice should convey reassurance.

Instead, the staff bombarded Sophie with verbal commands, none too gently delivered, such as, "Come on, Sophie, you know you are not allowed to be out here by yourself." "Let's go, Sophie! Now!" Most likely Sophie no longer even heard the content of these messages, but only perceived the tone of impatience and anger toward her.

5. Do not provoke the individual.

As if crowding around her, invading her space, and using harsh voices were not enough to frighten Sophie, several of the staff reached out attempting to grab her arm, presumably to take her back by force if she didn't comply with their commands. This action was the final trigger that escalated fear into panic and prompted Sophie to fend off what she perceived to be her attackers, by kicking and swinging her handbag at them.

In any caregiving institution where staff may be called upon to resolve conflicts involving emotionally fragile individuals, it is essential that caregivers have the skills necessary to accomplish resolution of conflicts through interventions that cause the least possible distress to all concerned, and to assure everyone's safety.

While the incidents involving Sophie were not life threatening, occasionally situations do arise in which an out-of-control person's behavior can result in serious injury to himself or others unless those who seek to resolve the conflict are trained in the techniques of nonviolent crisis intervention.

This particular staff not only lacked those skills; they failed to exercise the most basic courtesy and respect in their interactions with Sophie, thus violating her dignity and causing her acute emotional distress.

Every caregiving facility is responsible for the conduct and the quality of care given by their staff. It is flagrantly unfair to both the residents and staff when a facility fails to monitor staff performance and to assure that caregivers are adequately trained, and when it fails to increase staff competence by investing in further training as needed.

Most states require continued education for nursing home staff, and all of the facilities where I have worked complied with this mandate. However, having attended such programs, in most instances, I found the lectures to be too short and superficial to be of much value to the staff.

To be fair, most of the caregivers I worked with were dedicated and caring, but often did not have the skills to communicate effectively with their residents. And in nearly every facility, there were a few caregivers on staff who were not up to the requirements of the job.

I have great admiration for many of the nurses and CNAs it has been my privilege to know. The CNAs are the hardest-working caregivers in the nursing homes. They have the most intimate contact with the residents and perform the most difficult tasks. Yet they rarely receive praise or recognition for their efforts, and are often reprimanded for the smallest infraction. They are poorly compensated for their work, often earning little more than minimum wage.

It is a great failing of many nursing homes that when it comes to spending money and time on staff education, the CNAs are the ones most often neglected. It has been my observation that CNAs rarely, if ever, are given the privilege to attend seminars, such as the ones given by Mary Lucero, on Alzheimer's disease. If anyone at all is sent, it is usually the activity director, the social service director or a nurses supervisor. It is assumed that whoever is sent will pass on what they have learned to other staff in the facility, but in my observation that rarely happens. Yet it is the CNAs who are most in need of the opportunity to learn new skills that will help them in their work with the residents.

---

1. Mary Lucero, Lecturer: *Creative Intervention with the Alzheimer's Patient,* Videotape Lecture, (Winter Park, Florida: Geriatric Resources, Inc., 1992).
2. Crisis Prevention Institute. *Participant Workbook for the* Nonviolent Crisis Intervention® *Training Program.* Brookfield, WI: Crisis Prevention Institute, Inc., 2005.

To tell you the truth, feeding Paul is the most difficult thing I do all day.
—Lydia, CNA

Chapter 7

Paul was in an advanced stage of Alzheimer's. He was wheelchair bound; his limbs were severely contracted, his fingers bent into his palms, and his wrists twisted into an unnatural position. He could no longer turn his head, nor could his neck support the weight of his head, and he wore a neck brace to keep his head from flopping forward whenever he was seated in an upright position.

He could still chew and swallow soft food, although his appetite was poor. Like most Alzheimer's patients, he loved sweets and he was given a piece of cherry or apple pie for his midmorning snack.

Paul was brought to the dayroom at ten each weekday morning by his aide, Lydia, for his snack, and to attend the cognitive stimulation group I was leading at that time. Although he could not participate in any of the activities, we felt that he would benefit from the sensory stimulation he would receive by being in this social setting.

I had also incorporated midmorning snack time into my group. This strategy was helpful in getting some of the more restless and uncooperative residents to join the group—having been attracted by the goodies on the table, they were willing to sit down. Once they agreed to be seated, they usually stayed for the entire session as I engaged their attention with songs, games, and a variety of other activities. Some of the more alert residents enjoyed helping me serve their peers, and everyone had a good time.

The first morning Lydia brought Paul to the group, I could not help noticing that she had a great deal of trouble in her attempts to feed him his pie. He appeared to be startled each time the spoonful of pie touched his lips and Lydia encouraged him to eat by shouting, "Paul, open your mouth. Paul, you've got to eat."

Paul used his fists to push away Lydia's arm, and more often than not, he succeeded in knocking the spoon out of her hand. No amount of pleading on Lydia's part resulted in cooperation from him.

Once in a while, Paul opened his mouth to utter some guttural sounds, by way of protest, and Lydia was able to push a spoonful of pie into his mouth, which he then chewed and swallowed. But I could see that he was becoming more and more distressed, and Lydia's voice more strident, as her attempts to feed him continued to meet with resistance. Most of the pie ended up in Paul's lap, on his tray, and on the floor.

This scene was repeated the following day, and I was tempted to offer Lydia some advice. I had a fairly good idea why Paul reacted the way he did, and I knew there was a better way to get the nutrition into him. But I was reluctant to interfere in someone else's duties, and I was concerned that Lydia might interpret my attempts to help as criticism of her. Besides, I was very busy attending to my group, handing out cookies and drinks, mopping up spills, and assisting those who needed help.

I went to bed that night mulling over the problem Lydia had with Paul. I couldn't sleep until I had thought of a way to resolve this dilemma without offending her.

The following morning I commented to her that I had observed how difficult it was to feed Paul. "He really gives you a hard time," I said.

Lydia acknowledged that she was frustrated. She also expressed her concern that Paul was not getting enough nutrition. "To tell the truth," she added, "feeding Paul is the most difficult thing I do all day. I find it more exhausting than any of my other duties."

I asked Lydia if she would like to have a break from feeding

Paul his pie. I proposed that I take her place and feed Paul and she take over my job of serving snacks to my group. "That way we will both have a change from our regular routines," I said.

"Are you sure you want to do this?" she asked doubtfully.

I assured her that I did, and we traded places.

I had analyzed Paul's behavior from the perspective of the disease process, and I was fairly certain that his brain damage had progressed to the occipital lobe, which controls vision. In advanced AD, the patient's vision is damaged in very specific ways. It does not cause blindness, but it does destroy peripheral vision, and also results in what is called *downward restricted gaze*. Downward restricted gaze means that the person has lost the ability to move his eyes from side to side or up or down. In other words, the person's sight is fixed, or frozen, in one position. Given the fact that Paul also could no longer turn his head, I had to assume that his vision was now restricted to a very narrow field.

There is one peculiar phenomenon among Alzheimer's patients that relates to this vision impairment that does not manifest in persons with the same type of vision impairment who do not have AD. An Alzheimer's patient whose vision is impaired, as stated above, often does not respond to anyone who attempts to communicate with him verbally when that person is not within his field of vision, even if that patient's hearing is entirely normal. The Alzheimer's patient can hear the sound of a voice, but does not pay any attention to it, unless he can see the person who is speaking.

It may be that the stimuli of other voices and other noises in the environment all blend together in the person's perception and he cannot differentiate a voice that is addressed to him, and/or he may be distracted by other environmental stimuli at the same time.

This would also explain why one so frequently sees a startle response when someone touches an Alzheimer's patient without first having made eye contact with him.

That is why Paul flinched and became upset every time Lydia brought the spoon to his mouth. She was seated next to him, not in front of him, and thus was not in his field of vision. Paul did not see her, nor did he see the spoon coming.

Several days earlier, I had witnessed an incident with another resident who exhibited a startled reaction to being touched because she was unaware of the other person's presence. This resident was Norma, also an Alzheimer's patient in an advanced stage of the disease and, like Paul, confined to a wheelchair. She had been seated in the dayroom when two aides, India and Leslie, approached her from behind.

"Time to stand up for a minute, Norma!" Leslie sang out cheerfully as she and India came up on either side of the wheelchair, and each took hold of one of Norma's arms in an attempt to lift her out of her chair.

Norma led out a piercing scream that could be heard throughout the unit, as she shook off the hands of both aides. She banged the sides of her wheelchair with her fists, growling and muttering in acute agitation. The aides backed off and retreated several feet behind the chair.

I slowly walked up to Norma, smiled at her, and greeted her by name. Norma did not respond, nor did she make eye contact with me, but she stopped her growling and banging instantly, and reached out to the colorful long string of beads I was wearing. I came closer and bent down to let her touch them. Norma gently rolled the beads through her fingers, all the while cooing like a dove.

We stayed like that for several seconds. I bent down a little more to give more play to the beads in her hands. Now, for the first time, she made eye contact with me, and she gave me a dazzling smile.

It was then that I realized that due to downward restricted gaze, she had not been able to see my face when I was standing in front of her. All she had been able to see were my beads, which were at her eye level—in her field of vision.

When I explained downward restricted gaze and peripheral-vision loss to India and Leslie, they were skeptical, but when they followed my suggestion and knelt down in front of Norma so she could see them and hear them when they spoke to her, she willingly allowed them to lift her up to a standing position, and she took the required steps without protest while they supported her.

At this facility, getting wheelchair-bound residents on their feet for a few moments was to be done every two hours throughout the day to improve circulation and reduce seizing up of limbs. India explained to me that up to this point Norma had frequently reacted with hysterics and refused to cooperate, but in spite of that, the aides had been instructed to keep on trying. Needless to say, both aides were delighted with the success their new knowledge afforded them.

All this was on my mind as I pulled a chair up in front of Paul and bent low, so that I was looking up at him and was able to establish eye contact between us.

I greeted him with a smile and introduced myself by name. Of course, he would not remember my name or even my face once I left him. But it is important always to maintain appropriate social customs and amenities with any resident, no matter what his or her condition. One needs to take extra time when introducing oneself to a person with cognitive impairment, because such a person needs more time to process any new stimuli and to feel comfortable with a given situation.

Paul responded with a smile of his own, his way of communicating that he was pleased to see me. It is one of the greatest rewards of working with Alzheimer's patients that no matter how severely impaired they are, they appreciate attention and companionship.

I raised the plate with Paul's cherry pie in my left hand so that it came within his field of vision and told him what it was. "You like cherry pie, don't you, Paul?"

Paul's smile widened. I broke off a small piece of pie, and placed it on the spoon, keeping it in his visual field. I then asked him to open his mouth; at the same time, I opened my own mouth to cue him.

Paul complied, and only then did I bring the spoon to his lips. He chewed and swallowed without difficulty. I kept the plate and the spoon within his visual field at all times. After a few spoonfuls, Paul opened his mouth without prompting as the spoon with his pie traveled to his mouth. He ate the entire piece of pie in no time, and it was obvious that he had enjoyed it.

After the conclusion of my cognitive stimulation group, while Lydia helped me to straighten up the dayroom, she expressed her astonishment: "Paul never eats like that for me. How did you do this? Not even a crumb fell on the floor."

This was my cue to educate her about peripheral-vision loss and downward restricted gaze. Lydia was very receptive and tried this new approach at the very next meal she fed Paul. It worked as well for her as it had for me.

Lydia was a very caring person who often spent extra time with the residents assigned to her. Frequently she chose to spend an hour or more, after her shift ended, to do someone's nails, or play a game with them. But like so many other CNAs, she had just never been educated about the complexities of AD and how specific impairments affected the perceptions and the behaviors of the afflicted.

I am not suggesting that the behaviors of these patients are always predictable, or that specific strategies will always be effective in our interactions with them. On the contrary, the behaviors of Alzheimer's patients are more often unpredictable.

Neither am I suggesting that I knew with absolute certainty what Paul's perceptions actually were. But his reaction to Lydia's attempts to feed him had led me to believe that he perceived the situation as a threat.

Picture yourself confined to a wheelchair; your neck is in a brace and you can't move your head. Your hands are balled into fists that you can't open. You are unable to speak. You can see only what is directly in front of you, and what you see is confusing, You hear voices but you cannot understand them.

All you see of other people are legs and shoes passing in front of you at close proximity. You are feeling anxious, wondering where you are. Nothing looks familiar. All of a sudden, something gets shoved into your face. You can't see what it is. You don't understand what it means. Would you not feel threatened and afraid? Would you not fight this thing that keeps coming at you with all your might?

Judging by his reaction, there is little doubt that Paul experienced acute distress during Lydia's interactions with him. And for her the situation was equally distressing.

In contrast, a gentle approach, one that took into account his visual as well as his cognitive impairments, allowed Paul to experience his meal times as pleasant and safe encounters.

It is unfair to both the Alzheimer's residents and to the caregivers when the latter have not been educated about the specifics of the disease and have not been taught effective caregiving strategies.

Given the growing numbers of Alzheimer's residents in the nation's nursing homes, it is incumbent upon the management of these institutions to assure that their caregivers are adequately prepared to provide quality care for these residents.

I wouldn't give you away for a million dollars.
I never had a friend like you.

—Katie

Chapter 8

If one were to ask a CNA working with Alzheimer's residents which of their daily tasks they find the most difficult and stressful, most of them would probably say, "Bath time!"

That's because many of these residents tend to become fearful and agitated as soon as they are taken into the bathrooms. It is not unusual for them to become uncooperative and even combative with their caregivers. There are many reasons for these reactions, not the least of which is the environment of the bathroom itself.

Bathrooms in nursing homes do not look anything like the bathrooms people have in their homes. They were obviously designed for strictly utilitarian use, and no thought has been given to the feelings of the residents for whom they have been created. Even some of the alert and oriented residents dislike taking a bath or a shower in these rooms.

The impression one gets upon entering one of these bathrooms (they seem to be much alike in most nursing homes) is one of a cavernous, cold room that is cluttered with an assortment of equipment and furnishings that are positively bewildering. There are usually several outsized bathtubs, bath chairs with seats that look like toilet seats, and at least one Hoyer lift (used to lift the residents, stripped to the buff, from their wheelchairs into the bathtubs). Toilets and sinks are curtained off behind individual cubicles. To add to the clutter, the bathrooms in many facilities are often the place where extra wheelchairs are stored.

The monochromatic color scheme, most often a gloomy institutional green, only adds to the drabness of these rooms; there is not a single feature to attract the eye and nothing in the environment to give reassurance of a pleasant experience to come. Room temperature is often kept too low to be comfortable for a naked, frail elderly person. Caregivers are well acquainted with residents who struggle and fight every bath time in an attempt to avoid being taken into the bathroom. If the residents are forcefully taken (this happened routinely in all the facilities where I worked), they will continue to resist their caregiver's attempts to bathe them. By the time the bathing or showering is done, the resident may be totally traumatized and the caregivers may be nursing a few bruises. Staff dislike bath time almost as much as the residents do because it is very stressful for them as well. It is often difficult to complete the task in a manner that is safe for both the resident and the caregiver.

Anyone walking past a bathroom, during bath time, will almost always hear the screams of one or more residents and the loud cajoling voices of staff who are trying to reassure the residents that they won't be hurt, and pleading with them for cooperation. Even some of those residents who willingly go into the bathroom understandably become terrified if they are placed into the Hoyer lift, hoisted up, swung into position over the bathtub, and then lowered into the water. The ride itself can provoke panic.

In her lecture on Care of the Alzheimer's Patient, Mary Lucero has recommended that those residents who tend to become traumatized when given a bath or a shower should be given sponge baths instead.[1] This certainly seems to be the logical course to follow in order to spare the resident emotional distress. Yet I have rarely, if ever, seen this done.

Nursing homes, like hospitals, tend to do things the way they have always been done. They are very slow to change their established routines and procedures, even when there is absolutely no merit in holding on to some of these rules. Mary Lucero refers to "that big nurse in the sky who decreed how things are to be done."[2] It has always seemed cruel to me to force residents to endure procedures that are so frightening and emotionally destructive to them, when alternatives exist that would eliminate these problems.

In some instances, it is the caregiver's inappropriate approach to a resident that triggers a negative response at bath time. This was clearly the case when Alice, a new CNA on the Alzheimer's unit at the Willow Pond Nursing Home, attempted to give one of her assigned residents a shower for the first time.

According to the director of nursing (DON), Alice had never worked with Alzheimer's residents prior to being assigned to this unit. The DON explained to me that Katie, the resident who was to be given a shower by Alice, tended to be fearful of the procedure. "She always gives us a hard time," stated the DON, and it takes a lot of patience and persuasion before she is reassured and cooperates.

"But last night she became so enraged in the bathroom that she threw Alice on the floor and stomped on her. It took three people to pull Katie off her. And we had to abandon any attempt to give her a shower after that."

I was surprised to hear that; I knew Katie. She was in my cognitive and sensory stimulation group. The adjectives that came to my mind to describe her were warm, funny, cheerful, and sensitive to the feelings of others.

Katie was fifty-seven years old, of solid build, with rosy complexion, brown eyes, and short salt-and-pepper gray hair. According to her medical chart, she had been diagnosed with early onset of AD at age fifty-one. At the time of her admission to Willow Pond four years earlier, she had severe cognitive and memory impairments, but she continued to maintain good motor and language skills. Except for arthritis of the hip, she was in good physical health.

What I had learned about Katie in the several months I had been working with her was that she loved to sing, play dominoes, and water the plants in the lobby. She could recall and recite the ingredients for close to a dozen dishes she used to cook for her family. She remembered many of the hymns she used to sing in church, and she still sang these in a sweet soprano voice. Frequently that voice was the first sound I heard when I entered the Alzheimer's unit.

Yet Katie no longer recognized her son. When he came to visit her, she looked at him blankly. And when he reminded her, "Mom, I'm Danny. I'm your son," she shook her head and laughed.

"No, you're somebody else's son. My Danny is a little guy. He's in the sixth grade, you know," and she walked away from him. Once, her son brought in a photo portrait of himself as a child to help jog Katie's memory.

"Look, Mom," he said, as he held up the picture for her, "This was me, when I was a little boy, but I'm all grown up now."

Katie studied the photo and then grabbed it out of Danny's hand. "That's my Danny," she said, and then took the photo to her room, leaving her son standing there, alone once more.

During all the time I had known her, I had never heard Katie say a mean word to anyone. She was very protective of her peers. The only time I had seen her upset was when Edith, one of her best friends, got her hand caught in the spokes of her wheelchair and injured a finger. Katie got angry at the nurse who didn't want her to accompany Edith to the nurses' station, where Edith's wound would be cleaned and bandaged.

"Don't worry, Katie. I'll bring Edith right back to you," the nurse assured her. "Please wait here for her."

Katie stomped her foot and shouted at the nurse, "I'm coming because she is my friend, and I'm taking care of her."

Now the DON had called me to her office to ask me if I would talk to Alice and counsel her regarding appropriate approaches in caregiving for Alzheimer's residents.

"Unfortunately, she wasn't working on this unit when you gave your in-service on AD," she said.

"I would like Alice to give Katie a shower tomorrow evening.

She really needs it. But Alice is afraid that she won't be able to handle it," continued the DON.

"I can't spare anyone else to do it or to assist her. Besides, if Alice is to continue to work on this unit she has to learn how to work with these residents effectively. I have already talked to her myself, but since AD and counseling are your specialties, I thought it might help Alice if you talked to her."

Katie's shower was scheduled for seven the following evening. In the meantime, I spoke to Alice, who was still shaken by her last experience with Katie. She appeared to be relieved when I told her that I would assist her.

The following evening I went home to change into a drip-dry outfit and a pair of old sneakers. I was back at Willow Pond by six-thirty. Katie had just finished her evening meal, and I had half an hour to get her into a relaxed, positive frame of mind before it was time for her shower. She agreed to come for a walk with me, and I took her down to the pond to feed the ducks, an activity she particularly enjoyed.

At seven, we met up with Alice who was waiting for us in front of the bathroom. Katie stiffened and drew back as soon as Alice opened the bathroom door. She backed up against the wall behind us, shaking her head vigorously.

"I'm not going in there!" she screamed.

Alice was about to take Katie by the arm, but I shook my head and reminded her not to touch Katie and not to crowd her. I had warned her earlier that it was crucial not to lay hands on the resident, even in a friendly way, when that resident indicated that she is not pleased with what she was expected to do.

When I reassured Katie that I would go in with her, and stay with her, she reluctantly agreed. Once inside the bathroom, I guided her to one of the bath chairs, and Alice said, "Let's take off your clothes, Katie," and attempted to remove Katie's shirt. Katie balked and slapped at Alice's hands. Alice backed away.

I asked Katie if she would like to take her shirt off by herself. She nodded her head affirmatively and pulled her shirt off over her head in one smooth motion. She then permitted me to unsnap her bra and she removed that also. However, when I suggested she take off her pants, she absolutely refused.

I said, "Katie, taking a shower with your pants on won't feel very comfortable. I always take mine off when I take a shower."

Katie made no move to remove her pants. I waited to give her time to decide what she was willing to do. Finally, I asked her, "Would you like me to help you out of your pants?"

"No," replied Katie, "I can do it by myself." She pulled her pants down, but refused to step out of them. Both her sweat pants and her panties were bunched around her ankles as she sat down on the seat of the bath chair.

I asked her if she was comfortable that way and she replied that she was. She nodded her head in agreement when I asked her if she was ready for her shower. I then turned to Alice, who had been standing in readiness with the shower hose in her hands, and directed her to turn on the water.

As soon as the water began to cascade from the showerhead and Alice stepped closer to her, Katie's expression signaled apprehension, and she waved Alice off, screaming, "No! No! Please don't do it, don't do it, don't do it—it's too cold."

The water had not even touched her yet, but Katie was beginning to panic. I asked Alice to turn the water off, then turned to Katie and waited until she calmed down, which she did, instantly. Then I told her that we would let her decide when the water temperature felt just right to her.

I moved away from Katie and closer to Alice, directing her to turn on the water. As Alice did so, I held my hand under the spray and said, "Alice, it's too cold, make it warmer, please." Alice complied "That's much better," I said, then turned to Katie and asked her if she would like to test the water. Katie nodded; she put out her hand, and Alice moved a little closer with the hose, holding the showerhead over Katie's hand, and Katie said, "Yes, that feels good."

After that, Katie was relaxed and cooperative as Alice ran the water over her body. However, when Alice approached her with soap and a washcloth, Katie became instantly belligerent. "Don't you come near me with that, bitch, or I'll hit you."

Alice backed off a few steps, and there was a moment of tense silence as Katie glowered at us. Neither Alice nor I could anticipate what would happen next. It was clear that Katie was poised to use physical force to repel anyone from coming close to her. It was equally apparent that Alice was afraid of her, and Katie knew it.

I took the washcloth from Alice, held it out to Katie, and asked her if she would like to wash herself.

Yes, of course," replied Katie, still frowning. "I always wash myself, my mother taught me how to do it right."

She took the washcloth; I handed her the soap, and she washed herself very competently, while regaling us with a running commentary on how her mother had taught her to do it.

"She always said, 'Start with your face, then wash your neck—but don't forget to wash behind your ears—and use plenty of soap to get the dirt off.'"

She even kicked off her sopping pants from around her ankles and allowed me to wash her back and her feet—that is, after I had asked her permission to do so. She permitted Alice to rinse her off, after once more testing the water temperature with her hand.

She made no protest when Alice wrapped her in a towel and dried her (after asking Katie's permission). Katie was so relaxed now she was humming a hymn. Alice and I hummed along as we helped Katie into her nightgown and her robe.

Alice asked her, "Katie, would you like me to comb your hair, or would you like to do it yourself?"

"No, you can do it," replied Katie good-naturedly.

I knew that Alice had several other residents to get ready for bed, so I volunteered to take Katie to her room and put her to bed.

As I tucked her in, Katie grabbed my hand and said, "I wouldn't give you away for a million dollars. I never had a friend like you."

When I left her, I felt sadness for all the times Katie had to endure anxiety and helplessness because no one understood her needs or respected her feelings.

Before I went home that evening, I waited until Alice had all of her assigned residents bedded down for the night, then I asked her if I could join her for her break. I had some concern about how Alice had felt about my intervention with Katie. I worried that she might have resented it. When I expressed these thoughts to her, she assured me that she was glad I had been there to assist her.

"You can't imagine how scared I was to go back into that bathroom with Katie," she said.

She pulled up the right sleeve of her uniform blouse to expose a sizable black-and-blue bruise on her arm.

"See what she did to me? The bruises on my back are worse."

"Besides," she continued, "I learned so much from the way you interacted with Katie. I still can't believe how quickly she calmed down. See, it never would have occurred to me to let her test the water temperature, or even ask her if she wanted to wash herself. I didn't think she could do anything like that by herself."

Alice was thoughtful for a moment as she sipped her Coke. "But how did you know that what you said to Katie would work to change her behavior?"

"I didn't know," I admitted. "But I did know that if I could make Katie feel more comfortable about the situation, and give her some control, some choices, then her feelings and her behavior would most likely change for the better."

"By the way, Alice," I asked her, "could it be that the first time you tried to give Katie a shower you forgot to adjust the water temperature to a comfortable level before you wet her down?"

I hated to confront Alice or to embarrass her. But it was clear to me from Katie's remark that she anticipated the water to be cold.

"I don't remember, but it's probably true," Alice stammered. "Looking back on that first experience, I now know that I screwed up.

"I think I triggered Katie's anger the moment I opened the bathroom door. When she refused to go in, I just took her by the hand and pulled her in. Then, when she wouldn't let me take her clothes off, I scolded her and told her to stop her nonsense.

"By the time I turned the hose on I was so crazed by all the trouble she had given me that I just wanted to get the job done, and get us both out of there.

"As soon as I began to wet her down, she attacked me, knocked me to the floor, and stomped on me." Alice shuddered visibly as she recounted the experience.

Now I felt bad. I had wanted to be helpful and supportive to Alice. Instead, I had made her feel worse.

"You know, Alice," I told her, "We all have moments when we find it difficult to cope. Taking care of Alzheimer's residents can be very stressful. For you it must have been especially difficult. You were new on this unit. You had had no prior experience with these residents, and you probably were already tired and stressed by the time you took Katie for her shower."

"You have no idea how stressed out I felt," replied Alice.

"On the South Unit most of my assigned residents were alert and oriented. Most of them could perform their own ADLs (activities of daily living) with minimal supervision from staff. But even those who needed total care were usually cooperative.

"I used to have a good time with my residents. They shared their thoughts and feelings with me. If someone was depressed, or just in a bad mood, I could always cheer them up and make them laugh again.

"I loved my residents on that unit. There wasn't anything I wouldn't do for them—if I could. Don't get me wrong, I worked hard over there too. Alert and oriented residents can be very demanding."

I told Alice that I could appreciate how difficult it must be for her to adjust to working with the residents on this unit, given that they were all suffering from Alzheimer's.

"It isn't just difficult," replied Alice. "It was a shock to be suddenly confronted with residents who are all so seriously impaired. My experience on the South Unit was only with mildly demented residents. It was nothing like this unit. Caregiving is much more intense and time-consuming here. These people are not only confused and helpless; they have mood swings and behavior problems that I've never had to deal with before. One minute they smile, the next minute they assault you."

Alice looked angry and tense. I asked her what kind of training and orientation she had been given prior to her transfer to the Alzheimer's unit.

"Are you kidding," exclaimed Alice. "There wasn't any time for that. One of the CNAs on this unit left without giving notice. She just walked out and a replacement was needed double-quick to fill the position. I don't even know why I got picked. The director of nursing told me that if I didn't like it here, they'd hire someone else, and if I want to, I can go back to the South Unit.

"I've already told the supervisor that I want to go back as soon as they can get a replacement for me here."

I asked Alice what kind of assistance she has received from the staff on this unit to help her get oriented to her residents and her duties.

"On my first day here," Alice explained, "the unit supervisor reviewed the medical charts of my residents with me. Then she assigned me to work alongside Margaret (another CNA) so I could get to know my residents and learn the caregiving routines for them."

"And was Margaret helpful to you? Did she tell you about the individual personalities, any special problems, likes and dislikes of your residents?"

"In some respects, yes," replied Alice. "She told me that I would need assistance when doing cares for Eddie, Mathilda, and John, because they are resistant to cares. They get physical and hit us. She told me that Bridie cries a lot but to ignore it because it doesn't mean anything. She also told me that Katie is very stubborn and needs a firm hand."

I asked Alice, "How did Margaret interact with the residents during caregiving? Did she talk to them, smile or laugh with them, like you did with your residents on the South Unit?"

"Heck, no," replied Alice. She never talked to them, except to tell them to move a certain way or to hold still while she was doing cares for them.

"She did talk to Katie, but I think that's because Katie's a big talker. She asks a lot of questions and won't give up 'til she gets an answer. Margaret also yelled a lot at Henry to stop fidgeting or to let go of her arm. Henry likes to grab at anyone who comes near him, and once he gets a hold of your arm or your clothes, he hangs on for dear life and won't let go. Most of the time, you have to pry his hands off, one finger at a time. Margaret told me she's glad Henry isn't one of her regular residents. 'I hate grabbers,' she told me," Alice said.

I explained to Alice that Henry, most likely, doesn't let go because he can't. "His brain no longer signals his fingers to release their grip on whatever they're holding on to."

"I don't think Margaret knows that," said Alice. "She's convinced that Henry holds on out of spite. That's what she told me. 'Watch out,' she said. 'That Henry is as mean and spiteful as a devil.'"

I was appalled, not only at this CNA's behavior and attitude, but also that Alice had been given such an atrocious introduction to caregiving on the Alzheimer's unit.

I knew from personal observation that the majority of the CNAs in this facility were very caring and conscientious in their work and interactions with the residents. But unfortunately, in every one of the facilities where I worked there were a few nurses and CNAs whose attitudes and behaviors toward the residents were neither caring nor professional.

I asked Alice what she thought of the way Margaret had treated her residents.

"I didn't think she was doing a good job," said Alice, "I thought she should have been more gentle, more patient. I didn't feel comfortable with the way she treated them.

"But these residents are so different from the ones I worked with on the South Unit, and I have no experience with Alzheimer's patients. I didn't know what to think. And I'm having a real hard time with some of my residents. The other day Henry grabbed my uniform and nearly ripped it apart. It had such a big tear in it, I had to throw it away."

"There is an easy way to avoid Henry's grabbing at you," I told Alice. "Give him something to hold in each hand before you start taking care of him. That will keep him from trying to grab you."

"But what is there that I could give him to hold?" asked Alice.

"The safest, most practical items would be two small pillows made of terrycloth and stuffed with washable materials. You can easily make these yourself."

"Oh, you are so clever," exclaimed Alice. "How did you ever think of that?"

"It wasn't my idea," I told her "I saw this intervention being used at another facility, and it really worked well with a resident who behaved just like Henry."

A moment later Alice was serious again. "Gosh, I wish I had learned about AD before I came onto this unit. It's all just overwhelming."

"Didn't you have some education about it when you studied for your CNA certification?"

"Not that I can recall. That was more than five years ago. All I remember being told was that Alzheimer's causes dementia, that there is no cure for it, and that people die from it. I used to feel so good about the job I was doing on the South Unit," continued Alice. "Here I feel so unsure of myself. I feel that I still don't know enough about these residents and how to deal with them. They get upset every time they see me coming, and I don't know what I can do to change that. I feel so bad about it that I dread coming to work. That has never happened to me before."

Alice lowered her head in a gesture of defeat. When she looked up again, a moment later, there were tears in her eyes.

"Alice, the reason you feel so depressed is because you are a very caring person. As far as I'm concerned, caring is the most important quality a person needs to work with Alzheimer's patients. The rest can be learned, and I can help you with that—provided you will let me," I told her.

Alice wiped away her tears and blew her nose. "Are you sure you have the time for this?"

I assured her that it was not a problem. I suggested that it might be helpful for her to attend a few of the cognitive and sensory stimulation programs that I or a member of my staff conducted each weekday morning on this unit. I thought it would be a good way for Alice to get to know her residents in a different setting. It would serve to open her eyes to the numerous and varied skills and abilities many of these residents had retained in spite of their severe impairments.

I wanted Alice to see how alive, alert, fun-loving, and funny Alzheimer's residents could be. I wanted her to hear them giggle and sing and laugh and tease each other, recite poetry and share memories of long-ago childhood days. I wanted her to see their increased animation in response to the attention, affection, and stimulation we provided.

I wanted her to understand that, yes, disruptive and inappropriate behaviors did occur, occasionally. But I wanted her to know how quickly peace could be restored through positive interventions and reassurance, before the problems could escalate.

Alice could easily arrange to attend a few of our sessions, as she did not have to be on duty until three in the afternoon. And she showed up for the CSS program the very next morning. She joined us again the following two days. From her first visit, she began almost immediately to interact and participate in the program, and the residents responded warmly to her presence.

To assist her further in her desire to learn about AD, I lent her my videotapes of Mary Lucero's seminar entitled "*Creative Interventions with the Alzheimer's Patient.*"[3] These were the tapes that had been of such great value to me when I first began to work with Alzheimer's patients, and my staff had equally benefited from viewing them.

A week later, I was sitting in the tiny closet-office that had been allotted to our service by Willow Pond, working on a progress report for my supervisor, when Alice poked her head in and asked for a few minutes of my time.

Her eyes glowed with pride as she told me that she had given Katie a shower the previous evening.

"I used all the strategies you used with her last week and it worked just great," she gushed. "Katie was totally relaxed and cooperative the entire time."

"Congratulations," I said. "I knew you would do well."

"It is really amazing," continued Alice. "When I attempted to control Katie the first time I took her for a shower, it backfired, and I lost control, not only of Katie, but of myself as well."

"Now that I am giving her control—letting her decide how much she wants to do by herself, she is so agreeable. She even let me wash her hair.

"We sang her favorite hymns together while I lathered and rinsed her head. It was actually fun. I think Katie really enjoyed the time we spent together in that bathroom."

Alice paused for a moment. A frown appeared between her brows. She shook her head as if she were trying to shake off an unpleasant memory, then she continued.

"I used to think of my caregiving duties as doing things for and to my residents. Now I think of us more as a team, doing things together, to get done what needs to be done."

"That's quite a leap forward, I can see you have given it a lot of thought, and gained much insight. Bravo!" I praised her.

"When I first came to work on this unit I used to feel so tense, especially in the evenings, knowing how much I had to do to get my residents ready for the night. I never gave much thought to how they felt about the way I went about my caregiving chores with them.

"I thought, 'Well they're senile.' To me that meant they didn't understand anything. So it wouldn't matter if I talked to them or not.

"I hate to admit it, but I treated them just like Margaret did. I only talked to them to give commands, to tell them to hold still—move this way or that, lift their feet—while I undressed them cleaned, them up, changed them, and got them into their night clothes. The fact that they didn't cooperate with what I asked of them only confirmed for me that they are beyond understanding anything at all.

"Even after you demonstrated that my approach to Katie was the problem, that my attitude had caused her to assault me, I didn't get it about my other residents—I mean, that I had to change my attitude and my behavior toward them too.

"I thought, OK, Katie isn't all that senile, but the others are pretty far gone. Isabelle can barely get a full sentence out, before she forgets what she meant to say—Mathilda the same. Bob and Johanna babble nonsense. Bridie cries all the time. Henry grabs and mumbles. John repeats the same few words over and over, and Eddie and Irene are mute. And all of them were such a handful. I thought I would go crazy.

"It wasn't until I attended a few of your group sessions that I understood how ignorant and judgmental I was. It was a revelation to see how much more there is to each of these residents than I'd realized.

"I understand so much better what my job is all about. I'm a better caregiver now. I can tell by the way my residents respond. Now I talk to them all the time while I'm doing cares. I smile a lot, I sing to them, I tell them stories. Now I know that it doesn't matter if they understand the words. But they seem to understand from the sound of my voice and from my new attitude that I am a patient and kind person and that I will be gentle with them. Even Eddie, Irene, and Henry smile back at me. And Henry loves to hold his little pillows.

"Bridie doesn't cry so much anymore. All I have to do is give her a back rub, and talk to her softly, and she'll stop. All of my residents are more relaxed during cares. It used to take me forever to get done, because I had to spend so much time struggling with them. Oh, it's all so much better than it was."

Alice had barely taken time to breathe as she related her experiences and insights of the past several days to me.

"Bravo," I said again. "Alice, you are without a doubt the best student I have ever seen. I knew that you had all the qualities to become a great caregiver. You just lacked the knowledge needed to work with this population. I am so proud of you."

"Thanks," said Alice, "I have a surprise for you. I've decided to keep working on this unit. I have come to love my residents here, and I think they need me more than my residents on the South Unit."

"Wow!" I exclaimed, "That's wonderful, Alice. And I'm happy for your residents here on this unit, because I know you'll give them the best of care."

"That's not all," said Alice. "I've also decided to go back to school to get a degree in nursing. Maybe some day I'll be able to teach other caregivers about Alzheimer's disease and about good caregiving practices for these patients. I think a lot of caregivers need more education about Alzheimer's."

I told Alice I couldn't agree with her more.

---

1. Mary Lucero, Lecturer: *Creative Intervention with the Alzheimer's Patient*, Videotape Lecture (Winter Park, Florida: Geriatric Resources, Inc., 1992).
2. ibid.
3. ibid.

These are my treasures from home.

—Lillian

Chapter 9

Lillian was an attractive seventy-eight-year-old lady who navigated through the ravages of Alzheimer's disease with an indomitable spirit and a stubborn insistence on maintaining as much independence and autonomy as possible within the nursing home setting.

She had selective memories of her life. She could no longer recall the husband, now deceased, to whom she had been married for fifty years, nor could she remember that she had given birth to, and raised, three children.

She did have very clear and vivid memories of her childhood, her parents, and her siblings. And she clung to these memories by reciting them like a mantra, several times daily, to anyone who would listen—caregivers, housekeeping staff, peers, and visitors. Everyone who lived or worked at the nursing home had heard her story, some probably hundreds of time.

"You know, my mother died of pneumonia when I was only eight years old. She was laid out in the parlor and Daddy held me up so I could say good-bye to her. She looked so pretty in a blue dress with a white lace collar. She was holding a prayer book and a red carnation in her hands. I cried and cried when they took her away.

"My sister, Charlotte, who was the eldest, took over the household and the cooking. My daddy said we had to mind her and help out with the chores. There were seven of us, four boys and three girls. I was the youngest."

Lillian was able to describe her childhood home and the surrounding landscape in loving detail.

"Our house was very large. It had two stories, an attic, and a cellar. My favorite place was the porch. It ran all along the front of the house. It was glassed in so we could use it all year 'round. It had wicker furniture. I loved to sit there at the end of the day with my daddy to watch the sun go down behind the meadows.

"There was a small pond near our house where we went skating in the winter. Skating was one of my favorite things to do. Sometimes my hands got so cold inside my mittens that they felt like icicles. But I never let that stop me.

"In the summer, my daddy used to take us hiking in the woods. We picked wild berries and mushrooms. Daddy taught us which were edible and which were poisonous."

She reminisced about going to church with her father and her siblings every Sunday. "Daddy always lined us up in the parlor and inspected us to make sure we were clean and dressed in our best clothes, shoes shined, hair combed. He liked us to be neat and well behaved."

She remembered her father's kindness. "He never hit us, he never raised his voice. But when one of us had done something bad, he called that child into his study to decide on the punishment. My daddy didn't call it punishment; he called it consequences. Mostly, consequences meant not being allowed to go out to play after school. Once my brother, Jordan, had to stay in for a whole week because he had broken a window in the parlor and then lied, saying he hadn't done it. My daddy told him the lie was a lot worse than breaking the window.

"Mostly it was the boys who did bad things. I hardly ever got in trouble myself," declared Lillian. "I loved my daddy so much, I never wanted to displease him. I did get punished a few times, but I didn't mind having to stay in my room. I loved to be by myself to play with my dolls. But I was sad when I disappointed my daddy."

Whenever Lillian reminisced about her childhood, she used the exact same narrative, word for word. When someone interrupted her recitation with a question, she got flustered and confused, and she found it difficult to formulate a reply. She tended to stutter and mix up words. For instance, someone once asked her, "What kind of things did you get punished for?"

Lillian took a couple of deep breaths; a frown appeared on her forehead as she struggled to answer the question: "I . . . I . . . oh . . . I . . . let me think. I fiddle-daddled. No . . . fuddy-taddled . . . you know . . . when it was time to go to school . . . I . . . I . . . I . . . lost the bus."

Everyone present burst out laughing. Lillian covered her face with her hands. She sensed, I believed, that something was remiss in her reply, and she was embarrassed.

"I think Lillian meant to say that she dillydallied when it was time to go to school, and she missed the bus," I translated.

"That's it, that's what I said!" exclaimed Lillian.

In spite of the fact that Lillian enjoyed the attention she received from others, she was essentially a loner. She spent most of her time in her room.

According to caregivers, she had never set foot into the dining room in the six years since she had come to live at the Green Hills Nursing Home. She occupied a private room and ate all her meals there, at her request. She had consistently declined all invitations to come to activity/recreation programs or to join in the social gatherings with her peers. She would come out of her room two or three times each day to walk a few steps in either direction, then return to her room. On rare occasions she walked as far as the dayroom, but refused to sit down and socialize with her peers except to deliver her monologue about her childhood. She never showed the slightest interest in anyone around her beyond engaging their attention while she reminisced, and then abruptly leaving to return to her room.

As I came to know Lillian, I observed that she was very sensitive to an overload of stimuli. She simply could not tolerate the noise level generated by a group of people talking to each other, combined with the background noise of piped-in music and/or a TV program in progress. This sensitivity to multiple stimuli is a problem shared by many Alzheimer's residents. It is well known that these patients do best in a serene, quiet environment. However, few of them are able to retreat from the noises in the nursing homes as Lillian did.

Caregivers on her unit spent as much time as they could spare visiting her in her room, often bringing along one of the other residents, to encourage her to socialize. Lillian gave every indication that she enjoyed these visits, and she was consistently gracious and welcoming.

She was cooperative with caregivers, so long as their requests did not interfere with her self-chosen daily activities. She ate her meals when they were served; she took her medication when it was presented. She took her bath when directed, and she allowed her CNA to trim and polish her nails. She even consented to have her hair washed and set every other week, which required her to visit the beauty salon located on another unit. But she had low tolerance for any changes in her accustomed routines. She became hostile and verbally abusive with staff when she was asked to leave her room for any other reason.

When the housekeeping staff came to her room on their daily round of cleaning, Lillian, unlike most other residents, refused to leave her room, and the cleaning crew had gotten used to working around her. Lillian thought of them as her guests. She always greeted them warmly, often inviting them to sit down and take a rest. "You don't have to clean my room, honey. I can do that myself."

The housekeeping staff loved her and became so familiar with her stories from childhood that some of them could have recited them by heart.

However, at least once every three months, Lillian had no choice but to leave her room for several hours. It was on the day when housekeeping removed all the furnishings from her room, including the bed, in order to wax and polish the floor, wash the walls and windows, and change the curtains.

Most of the other residents were also unhappy when it was time for their rooms to receive a major cleaning. They grumbled about the inconvenience and fretted about their belongings. "They never put my stuff back the right way," they might complain. But then they cooperated and went off to the recreation programs or to sit in the dayroom while their own rooms received a thorough cleaning.

Lillian, on the other hand, refused to leave the scene of what she considered an outrage and a violation of the sanctity of her room. She followed the cleaning crew, berating and cursing them as they removed her furnishings from her room and piled them up in the hallway. Then she paced back and forth in front of the doorway, muttering to herself, harassing and threatening the cleaners. "I'll call the police if you don't hurry up and put my things back in there. You have no right to touch my things, you bastards."

Sometimes she became so agitated that she substituted or scrambled her words. I once heard her yell, "You . . . you flatbed baggers . . . I'm going to . . . to have you regrested! The pops will grain you . . . you'll see."

Caregivers took turns attempting to reassure Lillian that all her things would be put back into her room promptly, as soon as the cleaning had been completed. They tried to coax her to come away from the area, tempting her with offers to take her for a walk outdoors. They offered to let her make a phone call to one of her children from the nurses' station. But she would have none of it. She could not be bribed or patronized. Until her room was done and her furnishings were back in place, she regarded everyone on staff as her adversary. Once it was done, however, she calmed instantly and once more became the gracious lady everyone knew and loved.

When I visited Lillian in her room for the first time, I understood why she chose to spend so much time in it. The room itself was bright and spacious, with a large picture window providing a view of the well-tended lawn bordered by stately oak trees. An ornate fountain birdbath surrounded by a bed of flowers took up the center of the lawn.

The room was beautifully furnished with Lillian's "treasures from home," as she never failed to inform her visitors. Her bed was covered with an ivory crochet lace bedspread which provided a fitting background for the collection of needlepoint pillows that had been stitched by various members of her family. Above her bed hung a framed cross stitch sampler, created by Lillian's great-grandmother Ida Mae Gaebler in 1857. The name and date had been incorporated into the delicate floral design. Flanking the bed on either side were two dainty Chippendale tripod tables covered with lace doilies and matching pale blue glazed porcelain lamps with silk shades.

Opposite the bed, against the wall, sat a seventeenth-century, intricately carved walnut chest. Mounted above, a curio shelf displayed a collection of antique miniature dolls and clowns. Most of the rest of the walls were covered with framed group photographs and portraits of Lillian's extended family—parents, siblings, husband, children, and grandchildren.

A Queen Ann wing chair, covered in faded blue velvet, took up space in the left corner by the window. An unfinished crochet afghan, one of Lillian's current projects, was draped over the arm of the chair. A basket next to the chair held the yarn in three shades of pink.

The opposite corner by the window contained a tall mahogany bookshelf filled with old leather-bound volumes of classic literature, as well as Lillian's collection of contemporary novels and mysteries in large print editions. Lillian was still a prodigious reader, though she could no longer retain what she read.

Between the bookshelf and the carved chest sat a compact entertainment unit. The top held a TV and VCR. The shelve below contained an old-fashioned combination radio and record player. Lillian's collection of videos, mostly old movies from the 1930s to the 1950s, and her records of classical music were stored in the cabinet below. A wrought iron plant stand in front of the window, containing several well-tended pots of flowers, completed the furnishings in her room.

It was the most beautiful room I had ever seen in a nursing home. There was no other place in the facility that could compete with this environment of beauty, comfort, and warmth Lillian's family had created for her with her treasures from home.

She had her books, her music, her TV and VCR. She had a comfortable place to sit, with good light to read or to work on her crochet projects. She had her own private phone to keep in touch with her far-flung family.

Even though she did not participate in the group activities or entertainment provided for the residents, loneliness was not a factor. Despite the fact that she had been classified as a loner, she was not isolating herself. She enjoyed interaction with others, and she received daily visits from caregivers, peers, and housekeeping staff. At least once a week her youngest daughter, who lived about a hundred miles from the facility, came to see her. Other family members called her frequently. It did not matter that Lillian was oblivious of the caller's relationship to her. When asked who had called, her usual reply was, "Oh, that was one of my best friends"

I was requested to see Lillian initially because a major change was about to occur that would profoundly affect her lifestyle, and caregivers anticipated that it would be a traumatizing experience for Lillian. Karen, the social service director, filled me in on the details.

Six years ago, when Lillian's children had come to the painful decision to place her in a long-term care facility, they sold the parental home in the belief that the money from the sale, together with Lillian's modest savings left to her by her husband, would be sufficient to pay for a private room for their mother at the Green Hills Nursing Home, one of the best facilities in the area, for many years to come.

They had further assumed that in the event their mother's funds ran out, each of the siblings would be able to contribute enough cash to maintain her in her private room indefinitely. Although not wealthy, each of Lillian's three offspring was comfortable and financially stable at the time they met to discuss their mother's future needs and welfare.

They had not factored in inflation or the rising costs of health care, nor had they thought of the possibility that any one of them would suffer financial reverses, as had happened to the eldest son who had recently suffered severe financial losses in his business. Nor had they anticipated the steep rise in the cost of college education. Each of them had children, several of whom were currently enrolled in college, and others who soon would be. In short, Lillian's children were unable to contribute to her upkeep now that her funds were depleted.

Lillian had become eligible for Medicaid, which would pay the balance of her maintenance at the nursing home that was not covered by her monthly Social Security check. However, Medicaid did not cover the cost of a private room. Therefore, it had become necessary to move Lillian from her lovely private room to a double-occupancy room to be shared with a roommate.

This was going to be a most difficult adjustment for Lillian, for whom privacy was a major issue. Her personal space in a double room would be less than half the size of the large room she now occupied. Wall and floor space were too limited to accommodate more than a small part of her furnishings. Caregivers at Green Hills were extremely concerned about how this drastic change would affect Lillian.

I began to see Lillian two weeks prior to the official room change. My first objective was to gain her trust and her acceptance of me as a caring person she could count on when she was distressed. I began to visit with her several times per week. She always greeted me warmly and enthusiastically and went through the ritual of pointing out to me every item of furnishings and decorations in her room, explaining its provenance and its significance to her. She never remembered my name or who I was, but she treated me like a "dear friend" and introduced me as such to others.

"We went to school together, you know," she confided to those who saw us together as she put her arm proprietarily around my back.

She also consented to come outside to sit on the patio with me, or to go for a walk on the facility grounds. These were activities she had always resisted.

Lillian's new room had already been chosen. It was just two doors down from her present room, on the same side of the hallway. The view from the window was almost identical to the one she had now. She would not be deprived of watching the birds splashing in the fountain, one of her favorite activities.

Although she would eventually have to accept the presence of a roommate, the nursing-home administrator, on the recommendation of the social service director (SSD), had wisely decided to give Lillian time to get used to her new environment before the next element of adjustment, (the roommate) would be introduced into the situation.

In an attempt to prepare Lillian for the change, the SSD had discussed with her what was about to happen and why, but it was an exercise in futility. Lillian's mind could no longer process such complex information. She listened politely to the explanation from Karen, the SSD.

"Well, dear, I have a lot of money in the bank, so don't worry about me," Lillian stated, as she reassuringly patted Karen's hand.

When she was shown her new room, which was presently empty in preparation for a new paint job, and Karen asked her what color she would like to have it painted, Lillian replied, "I don't care, paint it any color you like. I have my own room and I like it just the way it is."

There was just no way Lillian could be prepared for the experience of a room change. All we could hope for was to prepare ourselves to provide as much emotional support as we could give her and, meanwhile, come up with a plan that allowed us to fit as many of her personal possessions as possible into a greatly reduced space.

At last the day of the move arrived. As arranged earlier that week I took Lillian to the hairdresser, who had been asked to take as much time as she could spare to delay Lillian's return to the unit. She even offered to do Lillian's nails free of charge in order to detain her a little longer.

After delivering Lillian to the hairdresser, I raced back to the unit to assist housekeeping staff, nursing staff, and the SSD in moving Lillian's belongings to her new room. While her bed was being made up and her furniture was moved in (as much as it was possible to place), I hung as many of her photographs and portraits as I could find room for. Whatever did not fit was whisked away to a storage room to be picked up later by Lillian's family. The tension was palpable among us as we speculated about Lillian's reaction to the move.

The room was done at last. As a final touch, the SSD brought in a vase of flowers and placed it on the bedside table, and I hung the decorative name plaque I had made for Lillian on the door.

When I picked her up at the hairdresser's a few minutes later, she was relaxed and cheerful, pleased with her nail polish and her newly set hair. She was oblivious of the significance of this day in her life, while I was mentally tortured with anxiety in anticipation of her reaction.

As we came down the hall of Lillian's unit, I noted with some relief that the door to her old room had been closed, and a linen cart had been strategically placed to obscure it.

Gently I maneuvered her past, chattering away at her, to further distract her from noticing her old room. In passing, I saw that several caregivers were hovering in the vicinity, trying their best to be unobtrusive, but obviously ready to be on hand in case Lillian should have a major meltdown. By unanimous agreement, the caregivers had designated me as the person to introduce Lillian to her new room, a dubious honor that I would gladly have relinquished to someone else.

The first thing Lillian took note of was the new sign with her name on the door. "Oh, that is pretty," she exclaimed. As I opened the door and guided her into the room ahead of me, she stopped for a moment on the threshold. She looked around the room with a puzzled expression on her face. Her eyes darted from object to object and finally came to rest on the second bed.

"How come there's another bed in my room?" she asked.

"Oh," I replied, "we thought it would be nice for you to have one. "Then, if you have a visitor, and the two of you would like to spend more time together, you could invite your friend to sleep over."

Lillian thought that over for a few seconds, then she smiled and said: "Well, you're a good friend. I'd like to spend more time with you. So how about staying over tonight?"

I had not anticipated that at all. For a moment I was speechless, my mind a blank. But I recovered quickly. I thanked Lillian for her kind invitation and asked for a rain check, pleading a previous engagement.

Her attention was already focused elsewhere. In fact, she now proceeded with her usual routine of familiarizing a visitor with the history of each of her belongings.

She pointed to her father's portrait, "That's my father; he was very kind, he never hit us he never raised his voice . . ." and she was off reciting her childhood memories.

Next she turned to the curio shelf, which had been mounted on the wall across from her bed, as in her old room. She explained, one by one, how she had acquired each of her miniature dolls and clowns. She pointed to the cross stitch sampler above her bed. "My great-grandmother stitched that." She invited me to sit in her wing chair. "That chair has been in my family for over a hundred years."

I knew that wing chair would have to go once a roommate took up residence in the other bed and needed equal space for her things. As Lillian recited all her oft-heard and very familiar memories, my tension mounted. Surely, I thought, any moment now she will notice that some of her furniture is missing, such as her carved chest, the second bedside table and lamp. She will realize that her entertainment unit is gone and her TV is sitting atop a much smaller shelf, which had been substituted for the one she had brought from home. Her old-fashioned record player had been replaced by a new radio/CD player that took up less space.

My mind was in turmoil as I braced myself mentally for a full-blown catastrophic outburst when Lillian realized that this was not her room. I also grieved for the new losses Lillian would have to adjust to. I empathized strongly with how painful these changes were going to be for her. I did not feel the least bit equal to dealing in a professional manner with the situation.

I glimpsed through the open doorway that several nurses and aides continued to hover in the hallway, ready to assist me when the moment of truth arrived for Lillian.

But she appeared not to notice any changes and was unaware of any losses. She did notice the new radio/CD player and picked up the note card her daughter had attached to it. She read it, then handed it to me.

"Isn't that sweet," she said, "Someone brought me this thing to play music. Will you show me how it works?"

I chose one of the CDs her daughter had sent, and demonstrated how to insert it and which button to push to activate it. Lillian expressed delight as the sound of music filled the room.

"That's the 'Moonlight Sonata' by Beethoven," she exclaimed. "It's one of my favorite pieces."

She sat down on her bed and invited me to sit next to her. While we listened to the music, Lillian's eyes continued to scan the room. For a moment, a tense expression crossed her face as she scrutinized the bookshelf.

"Here it comes," I thought, and braced myself for the explosion. But her eyes moved on to the picture window. Her face relaxed visibly as she spotted a couple of birds splashing in the fountain.

She spread her arms wide, taking in the room and the view.

"Isn't this nice," she declared. "I just love my room, don't you?"

It slowly dawned on me that the crisis had been averted and my tension began to melt away. Lillian appeared to feel perfectly at home in her new room.

After that, she frequently asked the staff why there was another bed in her room. The staff, following my lead, always told her it was there in case she wanted to invite one of her friends to sleep over. Lillian was always satisfied with that explanation, and it even served to get her to accept her roommate when one was eventually selected to share her room.

She continued to eat her meals in her room, and continued to refuse to attend any group activities. But she did consent to come out to sit on the patio with me, or to take walks through the facility's grounds whenever I visited with her.

Lillian also continued to pace the hallways several time, daily. During the next several weeks she often mistakenly stopped by her old room. But when she opened the door, and saw that it contained nothing familiar, she quickly retreated. Whenever she came back to her own room, or was directed to it by staff, and she saw the sign with her name on the door, and peeking in, recognized her treasures from home, she was reassured that all was as it should be.

As for myself and the caregivers on Lillian's unit, we had learned a valuable lesson from this experience. A concerted effort had been made by all involved to fit as many of Lillian's furnishings from home as could be accommodated into her new room. We had done all we could to recreate, though on a reduced scale, the environment of beauty and comfort to which she had been accustomed.

Nevertheless, we were positive that Lillian would notice the absence of some of her most prized possessions, and we had anticipated that it would take days, if not weeks, for her to accept her new room. We were sure that she would be traumatized by the change, and that her behavior would be erratic and difficult to deal with.

But Lillian surprised us all. When I first brought her to her new room, her attention had immediately become focused on what was there, *not* on what was missing. It was quite literally a matter of "out of sight, out of mind."

It has been my observation that patients with advanced AD, whose memories, thought processes, and attention span have been greatly diminished, tend to concentrate almost exclusively on the present.

Because so much has become strange, unfamiliar, and often terrifying for them, they tend to seek the familiar in any given situation. The familiar—be it objects, people, or a place they recognize—provides reassurance, and can be instrumental in restoring their emotional equilibrium.

In Lillian's case the new room contained enough familiar objects to reassure her that she was in the right place. Even though some of her favorite pieces of furniture were missing, the room was nevertheless dominated by the familiar. The view through the window was identical to the one she was accustomed to in her old room, thus reinforcing the notion that this was indeed her room.

But the major credit for the smooth transition of moving Lillian from her spacious private room to a double with half the space belonged to the administrator and the care team of Green Hills.

In all the years I have worked in nursing homes, I have never, before or since, witnessed such well-coordinated and cooperative teamwork between different departments of a facility.

The administrator, the SSD, the DON, nurses, aides, housekeeping staff, and even the beautician demonstrated sensitivity to Lillian's needs and feelings in the planning and execution of the room change.

When the time came to choose a roommate for Lillian, the same sensitivity and thoughtful planning were applied, taking into account Lillian's personality, interests, and preferences. The roommate was also carefully evaluated to assure, as much as possible, that she too would feel comfortable and be compatible with Lillian.

Mabel, the chosen candidate, also had AD, but was at a more advanced stage than Lillian. Although she could still comprehend most of what was communicated to her, she suffered pronounced aphasia, making it difficult for her to express herself verbally. Nevertheless, she continued to enjoy the companionship of others, and left it to them to do most of the talking while confining her responses to short comments, smiled, and nods of the head.

Like Lillian, Mabel had acute short-term-memory loss. She usually forgot, within minutes, all that was verbally communicated to her. Thus the stories Lillian repeated to her endlessly about her childhood and her "treasures from home" continued to be as new and entertaining to Mabel, as they had been the first time she had heard them.

Mabel could no longer perform her ADLs (activities of daily living) without cues and assistance. Left on her own, she would put her clothes on backward and/or inside out, or she forgot to get dressed at all before heading to the dining room for breakfast. Normally, the residents' assigned aides cued and assisted them with ADLs, as needed.

However, the staff assigned to Lillian and Mabel observed that Mabel's problems with dressing and grooming brought out the nurturing side of Lillian's personality. She appeared to enjoy helping Mabel to dress appropriately, reminding her to brush her teeth, even showing her how, and she performed such additional services as brushing Mabel's hair, putting on her shoes, pulling up her socks, and buttoning her sweater or blouse—all chores that had become too complex for Mabel to do for herself. Mabel accepted Lillian's ministrations good-naturedly.

Wisely, the staff assigned to supervise and assist with ADLs refrained from interfering, as they realized that both Lillian and Mabel derived pleasure from their interactions. It was a symbiotic relationship that served both residents well.

Before long, Lillian introduced Mabel to others as her "sister," and Mabel referred to Lillian alternately as her "mother" or her "best friend."

Mabel, being the more passive of the roommates, but also more willing to accept guidance from staff, was picked up each morning and afternoon by Evelyn, the recreation aide, who escorted her to scheduled programs.

Evelyn never failed to invite Lillian to join them. But Lillian continued to decline, preferring to engage in her customary, solitary pursuits: reading, watching TV, or listening to music. When Mabel was brought back to their room, Lillian greeted her like a long-lost friend "Where have you been, honey? I missed you so much." And Mabel invariably replied, "I missed you too," as they hugged each other.

Then, less than a month after Mabel and Lillian had become roommates, the unexpected happened—thanks to Mabel. One morning, Mabel asked Lillian to come with her to the recreation room; she asked but once, and Lillian immediately agreed to go.

For years, ever since Lillian had been admitted to Green Hills, the staff involved in her care had encouraged her to attend and participate in the recreation programs in the belief that she, like most other residents, would benefit from the stimulation these programs offered and from the companionship of her peers. Every sort of enticement had been used, short of coercion, to tempt Lillian to come to the programs. "You will have fun, you will make friends. We are baking cookies today. There will be entertainment . . ." Nothing worked; Lillian could not be persuaded.

And yet, with just one request from Mabel, Lillian agreed to attend. What made the difference in Mabel's approach? She did not promise Lillian that she would have fun. Nor did she use any other lures designed to assure Lillian that coming to the program would benefit her in any way. Mabel simply said to Lillian one morning, "Oh, deary, please come, I need you."

I NEED YOU—the magic phrase that would have motivated Lillian to go to the end of the earth with Mabel, if she asked her. The need to be needed, to be of assistance to others, was very pronounced in Lillian at this time in her life, and she always responded to it, not only with Mabel but with anyone she perceived as needing support.

Any person placed in a nursing home will go through a period of adjustment.
Some people will go through a more intense period than others.
Some people will not make the adjustment.

—Doug Manning
The Nursing Home Dilemma[1]

Chapter 10

Being admitted to a nursing home is a time of great stress and anxiety for almost every person who undergoes the experience, not only because the event is usually preceded by debilitating illness, but also because it signifies a total break with all that the person has known and cherished. The cumulative losses of one's independence, one's home and belongings, one's accustomed daily routines and interactions with family and friends, as well as the loss of privacy, are traumatic for almost everyone who faces this situation.

Even if the person knows and understands that he can no longer function on his own, he rarely finds it to be a consolation that his needs will now be taken care of by others, because in addition to all the losses he has suffered, he will have to adjust to a whole host of rules and regulations that will govern his life from now on.

The new nursing home resident will have to become accustomed to three different shifts of caregivers attending to his personal needs within every twenty-four-hour period. In spite of the fact that upon admission he will be asked to state his personal preferences as to the kind of food he likes, what time he prefers to go to bed and arise in the morning, and whether he prefers to take a shower or a bath, in the morning or in the evening. In reality, in most nursing homes, he will have to eat his meals and take a shower or bath and go to bed, not when it suits him, but at specific times controlled by the institution. He will have to get used to a narrower choice of food than he may be accustomed to and to food that is usually more bland than he finds palatable. And if he has been used to eating lots of fresh fruits and vegetables, he will be out of luck at most nursing homes. He will have to get used to eating his meals in a room full of people and listen to near-constant piped-in music that would likely not be the kind he would choose to listen to. In many nursing homes this music is frequently interrupted by the public address system used by the staff throughout the day to page or to relay messages to each other. As he walks down the hall to and from his room, additional noise will come at him from the TV sets in individual rooms, some of which are on all day long. Unless the new resident is financially well-off and can afford to pay for a private room, he will have to share a room with another resident.

Nearly all newly admitted residents initially experience anxiety and depression. Such feelings can intensify and become chronic unless the person receives adequate attention, emotional support, and reassurance during the first several days after admission, and for as long as it takes to help him adjust to his new environment and the routines of the institution.

In most nursing homes in the United States it is the responsibility of the SSD to monitor the emotional well-being of the residents. The SSD is trained to recognize mental health problems and is expected to take appropriate action to assure that residents who exhibit signs of such problems are seen by a psychiatrist who will, in most cases, prescribe antidepressant or antianxiety medication.

However, what newly admitted residents need most of all is someone to spend time with them, someone who is a good listener, sensitive to their feelings, their anxieties, their fears—someone they can count on for emotional support on a sustained basis. Ideally this person will have the skills to assist the depressed person in helping him articulate what troubles him most. This person will not only help him to adjust to his new environment and situation, but will also take the time to introduce him to some of his peers, encourage him to socialize and to participate in recreational activities in the hope that some of these may engage his interest and serve to decrease the new resident's ruminations about his losses.

There are many caring nurses and nurses aides who possess the skills and the compassion necessary to fill that role successfully. Unfortunately, many nursing homes are seriously understaffed, and caregivers are hard-pressed to provide basic care for their assigned residents. They simply do not have the time needed to console and reassure a depressed resident. In recent years, this staff shortage has been getting progressively worse.

There is general agreement among health-care professional that a holistic approach to caregiving is the most effective route to healing and to the well-being of their patients. With the marginal staffing one encounters today in most of our long-term care institutions, caregivers are, in effect, denied the privilege to practice their craft as it was meant to be practiced. Instead, they are forced to provide care for the maximum number of patients in the shortest possible time.

It seems then that it is left to the residents' families to provide emotional support when a loved one is having a difficult time with adjustment. Yet family members are rarely effective in that role. Families often feel a great deal of guilt when they have to place a parent or a spouse into institutional care. They may find it too stressful to cope with their own feelings to be of much support to the new resident. In other cases the family may not have the kind of close relationship with the person that would allow them to share their feelings with each other. Or they may simply be too busy to visit with the resident more than briefly or sporadically.

In some cases a resident may be reluctant to talk to a spouse or a child about his emotional distress. A resident once confided to me, "I don't feel I can talk to my daughter about how unhappy I am here, because if I do, she may not want to come to visit me anymore. And that would be the worst thing that could happen to me. So I try to be cheerful when she comes."

Such fears are not always unfounded. As one family member explained her decision to visit her mother less frequently, "I get depressed every time I visit my mother. It's just too painful for me to listen to her constant complaints about having to live here. She asks me every time I visit her, 'Why can't I live with you?' It makes me feel terrible. She doesn't understand that the demands of my job, my children and the household use up all the energy I can muster. I just can't take on the additional responsibility of her care."

Most families at least try to visit with their loved ones in the nursing homes on a regular basis. Many bring special treats from home, a potted plant or a bouquet of flowers to brighten the resident's room. They bring cookies, fresh fruit, or even a home-cooked meal now and then. Some families take the resident out for lunch at a restaurant, once in a while, or for a shopping trip to a mall. Some even take the resident home for a day or two during the holidays, if it is practical to do so. Most of all, these families maintain their connectedness with the resident. There is no doubt that the continuity of familial relationships contributes significantly to the well-being of the residents.

During the years I worked in nursing homes, I have witnessed incredible acts of devotion by family members of nursing home residents. One such person I recall with great admiration is Kevin O., who came to the nursing home every single day to spend time with his wife, Katherine, who had Alzheimer's disease and was severely impaired. Not only did Kevin spend the entire day with Katherine, he actually took care of her every need.

He usually arrived at the nursing home early in the morning, gave his wife a sponge bath, dressed her, brushed her teeth and her hair, and fed her breakfast. Then he took her out to the patio in her recliner chair and sat with her until it got too hot for comfort out-of-doors. During the cooler season, he often fed Katherine her lunch on the patio as well.

Since I often retreated to the patio to write progress notes for my clients' medical charts, I had many opportunities to observe

Kevin with Katherine, and I was awed by the patience and tenderness he employed in all his interactions and ministrations with her. Often he massaged her hands or stroked her brow, or changed her position in the recliner, all the while talking to her as if she could still understand what he was telling her—and maybe she could—because her eyes never left his face. He even prepared her for bed in the evening and waited until she was asleep before he went home. No one at the nursing home received more tender loving care than Katherine did.

I once expressed my admiration to Kevin for the time and effort he devoted to Katherine's comfort. He told me that Katherine had married him after the death of his first wife, when he had been left with three young children to raise.

"I did not love Katherine when she agreed to marry me," Kevin stated. "I hardly knew her at the time. You see, it was an arranged marriage, suggested by my aunt Gertie, who convinced me that the children would be better off with a stepmother than just a dad. Katherine agreed very reluctantly to become my wife. She had just been jilted by a fellow, shortly before they were to tie the knot, and she wasn't ready to place her trust in another man. If it hadn't been for my aunt Gertie and her uncle Matt, it never would have happened. Those two plotted to get us together and practically pushed us to the altar."

Kevin took Katherine's hand in his and patted it gently as he continued to tell me about their life together. "I know this will sound like a fairy tale, but the fact is that Katherine was such a good wife to me and a wonderful mother to my children, that it didn't take long for me to fall in love with her. And I still am in love—even now." Kevin paused while he repositioned Katherine in her chair. Then he picked up her hand again and held it as he continued.

"Katherine and I had many interests in common. We both loved country music, playing golf, hiking. We loved to travel and explore new places. While the children were young, we rented a trailer during summer vacation and traveled out west to New Mexico, Arizona, California, up the coast to Oregon, Washington, and north to Canada. After the kids were grown and on their own, we went to Europe, the Far East, South America. We had twelve years of travel and adventures together before Katherine got sick." Kevin shook his head. "This Alzheimer's is one lousy deal. She doesn't deserve this."

When I asked Kevin where he found the strength to care for his wife, day after day, without a break (he had been doing it for the past eight years), and pointed out to him that this nursing home had excellent caregivers, he replied, "What else would I be doing? Katherine spent years taking care of me and my children. I was a wreck at the time we married. Katherine quite literally saved my sanity. She was the best companion any man could ever hope for."

It was obvious to all of us who worked at the nursing home that the daily care of his wife was taking its toll on Kevin's own health, and everyone tried to convince him to take time off for a rest. One day when he appeared to be especially tired and dispirited, I suggested that he should take a break, do something he enjoyed, and let the staff take care of Katherine for a few days. Kevin admitted that his physician had told him the same thing. He mentioned that he had been thinking about taking a few days off. He had traveled with Katherine all over the world, but he had never been to New England, and since the fall colors in that area were about to hit their peak, he decided to take a trip there.

Everyone at the facility applauded his decision. With the good wishes of the nursing staff for a pleasant journey, and their assurances that Katherine would be well taken care of during his absence, Kevin got into his car and headed north to New England.

A few days later, to my surprise, I found Kevin sitting on the patio with Katherine at his side. He told me, with tears in his eyes, that he had gotten as far as Connecticut, driving along, listening to their favorite music on the radio and enjoying the beauty of the fall colors when he thought about how much Katherine would have loved to share this trip. He was overcome by such profound sadness for the loss of her companionship that he felt it would be too painful for him to continue. So he turned around and came back to Florida to be with her.

Kevin's devotion to his disabled wife is unusual and quite extraordinary. At the other extreme are those residents who do not have a single surviving family member or even a friend, and there are more of such residents than one would expect. These residents seldom if ever receive visitors, and are therefore most in need of individual attention from nursing home staff.

These are also the residents who tend to have the most difficult time adjusting to the nursing home. This is particularly true when the nursing home staff has failed to spend extra time with them immediately upon admission and in the first crucial days afterward, when they feel most anxious and apprehensive about their new environment.

Yet it happened all too frequently that when a new resident was admitted who was not accompanied by a family member or a friend, he was often abandoned in his room for long periods of time before someone on staff found the time to attend to him. Such treatment was particularly frightening to those who were confined to bed or to a wheelchair and could not leave the room to seek help. Not even shortage of staff can justify such cruelty.

---

1. Doug Manning, *The Nursing Home Dilemma*, (Oklahoma City, OK, Insight Books, Inc., 1985), 54.

Not candy . . . not cake . . . no, no, that other thing . . . you know.
—Helene

Chapter 11

Helene was a new resident who had been at the facility less than a week when the DON asked me to see her. She informed me that since Helene had been admitted she has been spending most of her time in her room, crying. Sometimes she cried quietly, barely making a sound; other times she howled in a loud voice that disturbed the entire unit. She has not been eating well and has not been cooperative with caregivers.

"This appears to be more than a problem of adjusting to her new environment," added the DON. "We think Helene is clinically depressed and in need of treatment."

Before going to see Helene, I read her medical chart, as was my custom, to familiarize myself with her medical and social history. According to the information contained in her chart, Helene was recovering from a hip fracture. At her admission she had also been suffering from dehydration. She had had a mastectomy in 1985, but was currently free of cancer. She also had a diagnosis of AD with severe cognitive impairment. She could communicate verbally in a limited way, primarily by answering closed-ended questions with "Yes" or "No."

Her social history provided the following information: She was born and raised in a small town in Pennsylvania, the only child of immigrant parents from Ireland. She never married. She worked her way through teachers' college and then taught in New Jersey public schools until her retirement in 1976, at the age of sixty-two. She then worked part-time in a day care center until she became ill with breast cancer at age sixty-eight.

Helene had been living alone until that time, but now moved in with a friend who took care of her. Although the mastectomy was successful in removing the cancer, Helene was never completely well from then on. Since she had no living relatives, her friend continued to care for her after Helene was diagnosed with Alzheimer's disease, almost five years ago. In recent months her condition had deteriorated, and her latest fall resulted in a fractured hip. Helene's friend felt she could no longer care for her, and had admitted her to the nursing home.

When I arrived at Helene's room, I found her sitting in a wheelchair by the window. Her shoulders were hunched over and she was crying; actually it sounded more like whimpering. She did not respond to my greeting but continued to cry. I noticed that she was dressed in a flimsy sleeveless house dress with buttons down the front. Her dress was so short that it did not cover her knees. The two lowest buttons were missing, thus exposing most of her thighs. She wore neither stockings nor socks, and on her feet she had the kind of slippers that had a wide band across the top, so that most of her feet were exposed.

The room was frigid with the air-conditioning unit humming right next to where Helene was seated. When I touched her hands they were ice cold, and the fine hairs on her arms were literally standing up. It was immediately apparent to me that Helene was chilled to the bone.

"Helene," I said, "You are feeling very cold, aren't you?"

She did not respond, but continued to cry. It occurred to me that because of her advanced dementia, she could not verbalize her discomfort; she probably could not even conceptualize to herself the cause of her discomfort.

When I attempted to turn down the air-conditioning unit, I found that the knob was missing. I could not turn it off as that function was controlled inside a locked plastic box mounted on the wall by the door.

"Helene, I am going to make you feel better," I said, as I opened her closet door to look for a sweater. I did not find one. Her closet contained only more of the same kind of flimsy garments as the dress she was wearing. I did find a large afghan in a dresser drawer. I pulled it out and covered her with it from head to toe.

I gave her a gentle rubdown to speed up warming her body, and within minutes, she stopped crying. When I asked her if she felt better, she nodded her head in the affirmative and smiled. "Thank you," she said.

I gave her a hug and told her that I would be back shortly with a warm drink and a snack. "Would you like coffee, tea, or warm milk?"

"Coffee," she said and added, after a pause, "Can I have a sweet? Not candy . . . not cake . . . no, no, that . . . that other thing, you know." She was grasping for the right word, but could not retrieve it.

"Is it a cookie you want?' I asked. "Yes, yes, a cookie," she shouted and clapped her hands together, so pleased that I had understood.

"I will bring you two cookies and coffee," I promised.

Helene threw me a kiss as I left the room. When I returned with her refreshments a few minutes later, she looked at me, she looked at the tray in my hands, then she began to howl, her whole body convulsed with wracking sobs. Tears flooded her eyes and spilled down her cheeks.

I was flabbergasted—I was alarmed. "Helene, what's wrong?" I put down the tray, knelt beside her, and put my arms around her. "What happened, you were so cheerful before I left. What is making you so sad?"

Helene stopped crying, as instantly as she had started. She wiped her eyes with the edge of her afghan; she shook her head. "Not sad—glad, so glad." She pointed at me. "You," she pointed at the tray, "this coffee, the—not candy, you know."

"You mean the cookies?"

"Yes, coffee, cookies—you. So good, so nice."

"You mean you were crying just now because you feel happy?"

"Yes, happy, so happy." Helene grasped one of my hands and held it to her breast as her tears began to flow once more. "Thank you," she said.

I was so moved by her reaction to the simple, basic comforts I had provided that my own eyes were tearing up. Now we were both crying.

"Listen Helene," I said. "We have to stop crying. Your coffee is getting cold," and I set up the tray table in front of her.

I spent another half hour with her to solidify the rapport we had established and to get to know her better. She did have serious cognitive impairments and pronounced aphasia. Although she appeared to comprehend most of what was communicated to her, she had great difficulty expressing her thoughts verbally. I felt she would benefit greatly from participation in the cognitive stimulation group and from socializing with her peers. I was looking forward to doing a full assessment of her, and to including her in the MHNH program.

After I had reassured Helene that I would visit her the following day, I left her to speak to the DON. I reported my observations of the problems I had encountered and recommended that more appropriate clothing and footwear be obtained for Helene (the DON had been unaware of the lack thereof). I also recommended that the temperature of Helene's room be adjusted and checked on regularly.

I wish I could state that the caregiver's failure to note this resident's discomfort resulting from inappropriate attire and a frigid room was an isolated incident. Unfortunately, it happens all too frequently. I could not begin to count the number of times I have had to go back to the units to gather up sweaters and afghans for residents who had been brought to my group programs and felt cold because they had not been appropriately dressed. This failure to take prevailing temperatures into account when dressing a resident was a problem at every facility where I have worked. Consideration must be given to the chill caused by air conditioners, or the time necessary, during a cold snap, for the heating systems to warm up the buildings.

Nurses and aides are busy people. They move around at a brisk pace all day long in the performance of their duties. They are, generally, younger than the residents, and it can be assumed that their blood circulation and homeostasis (metabolic adjustment to temperature) are within normal range.

In contrast, older people, especially those who live in nursing homes, tend to be frail and much less active, and many of them are confined to wheelchairs. They suffer from a variety of debilitating diseases, and a large number of them have poor circulation. These residents need to be more warmly dressed than the average person to maintain their levels of comfort.

An Alzheimer's patient who has suffered severe brain damage, as in Helene's case, most likely has a damaged hypothalamus, and therefore lacks the internal controls that regulate body temperature. Mary Lucero, in one of her lectures on AD made the statement: "A resident with advanced Alzheimer's disease is the coldest person on your unit."[1]

To compound the problem for Helene, she was unable to walk, due to her recent hip fracture. Therefore, she did not get any exercise, which might have helped in keeping her body temperature at a more comfortable level.

Yet another problem that prevails in many of the older nursing homes, where buildings are often thirty years old, or more, is that the temperature tends to fluctuate from unit to unit, sometimes even from room to room.

Helene's attire the day I met her was completely inadequate and inappropriate given the temperature in her room and her general condition. It was inexcusable. OBRA states clearly that nursing home caregivers must *anticipate* and meet the needs of the Alzheimer's residents who can no longer judge or verbalize their needs.[2]

The next several days confirmed what I had suspected the day

I met her: Helene was not clinically depressed. Once she was appropriately dressed and her room temperature had been adjusted, her behavior changed dramatically. She was no longer crying. She was taken to the dining room for her meals and her appetite improved. Her physician approved her inclusion in the MHNH program. After that, it was a joy to watch her adjust to life at the facility. She even regained some of the verbal skills everyone had assumed she had lost, and before long, she had made friends with several of her peers.

When Helene was admitted to the facility, the staff had failed to make her feel welcome and to make certain that she felt comfortable in her room, to assure her that her needs would be met, to bring her out of her room, regularly, to introduce her to her peers, and to familiarize her with the facility, with the daily routines and with the services offered to the residents, such as the recreation programs and the dayrooms where residents gathered to socialize.

And even if Helene had shown no interest in anything or anyone, someone should have been assigned to look in on her and spend time with her on a regular basis during the first critical days after admission. Instead, she was abandoned in the worst possible condition, in a room that was too cold, inappropriately dressed, physically uncomfortable, lonely, and depressed. There is no excuse for such treatment of anyone, but it is especially unforgivable when perpetrated on a frail and emotionally fragile person.

---

1. Mary Lucero, Lecturer: *Creative Intervention with the Alzheimer's Patient*, Videotape Lecture (Winter Park, Florida: Geriatric Resources, Inc., 1992).
2. OBRA (Omnibus Budget Reconciliation Act), The Nursing Home Reform Legislation enacted by the U.S. Congress in 1987 and implemented in 1990.

The facility must promote care for residents in a manner and in an environment that maintains or enhances each resident's dignity and respect in full recognition of his or her individuality.

—Quality of Life
Federal Regulations[1]

Chapter 12

Theodora had been a nightclub entertainer in her native New Orleans, Louisiana, when she was young. It was the period in her life she remembers best, and her eyes sparkled whenever she talked about it, which she did often, with anyone who was willing to listen.

Reminiscing was not all she did. Now, at age seventy-five, she could still sing her heart out; she could tap-dance; she could do an impressive high-kick, and she was determined to use every opportunity to demonstrate her talents to her fellow residents and to the caregivers at the Sunny Hill Nursing Home.

Although her glamorous career was nearly half a century in the past, Theodora still craved the attention and the applause she had once received for her performances. The problem was that due to the brain damage of AD, she could not remember that she was no longer in show business.

Whenever the nursing home provided entertainment programs for the residents, Theodora could not resist participating in the event. Frequently, she disrupted the performers in the midst of their routines. It did not matter if it was a solo performer or an entire chorus of singers, Theodora would simply walk onstage and, with a grand gesture, wave the entertainer aside, grab the microphone, and belt out one of her nightclub songs, some of which tended to be a bit raunchy. On several occasions, in the midst of his service, she had even interrupted the priest, Father John, from St. Agnes Parish, who came once a week to say Mass for the Catholic residents.

Most of the entertainers, as well as Father John, were tolerant and understanding of Theodora's antics. Not so her peers. They became enraged and hostile, shouting and booing and calling her vile names. Some even threatened to beat her up, and a few actually succeeded in following through on those threats. Sometimes it became necessary for staff to remove her quickly from the area for her own safety.

Theodora's reaction to these outbursts of hostility from her peers were shock, humiliation, and tears. She could not understand why her performances were not appreciated, and it required much effort from caregivers to console her.

To prevent such incidents, the staff told Theodora in advance of scheduled entertainment that it was not appropriate for her to interrupt the performers. And they extracted a promise from her that she would behave and sit quietly until the program ended. Of course, this strategy met with complete failure. Although Theodora was a considerate person who was anxious to please and willing to abide by rules, she could not comply because within five minutes of giving her promise not to interrupt, she had already forgotten about it.

Her love of performing, singing, and dancing was still such an intrinsic part of her personality that she simply had to express it as often as possible. She not only disrupted formal entertainment, her compulsion to entertain was triggered any time she came upon a group of people. Regardless of whether there were three or four or twenty gathered together, be it in the dayroom, the visitor's lounge, the recreation room, or even on the patio, Theodora could not resist putting on a show.

She carried a long diaphanous scarf in the pocket of her dress, and sometimes she whipped it out and swirled it about her dramatically, while treating her audience to one of her performances.

One of the nurses once commented, "We must be thankful that Theodora was not a stripper. Can you imagine how shocked some of the ladies would be if she were to take off her clothes as part of her act?"

"On the other hand, just think how the men would love it," retorted another.

Some of her peers simply ignored Theodora's impromptu performances, but the majority of them were not amused when she interrupted them while they were watching TV or playing cards or engaged in various other activities that required their concentration.

Theodora was subjected to daily verbal abuse and sometimes even a push or a slap from her more aggressive peers. Several of them had come to dislike her so much that as soon as they saw her approach, they shouted at her, "Get out of here, get lost. You better not bother us with your stupid song and dance routine." and other similarly hurtful remarks.

Caregivers had to spend an inordinate amount of time, almost daily, intervening in these altercations to prevent them from escalating to more serious confrontations and to protect Theodora from further abuse. They constantly sought ways to prevent the hostilities between Theodora and her tormentors. They had even, at one time, implemented a behavior management plan designed to reduce or extinguish Theodora's compulsion to perform. But they had been unable to make it work.

The obvious resolution would have been to keep her physically separated from those of her peers who could not tolerate her intrusive behavior and had developed an aversion to the mere sight of her. But such separation was not feasible in this facility.

Sunny Hill was one of those nursing homes that accepted alert and oriented residents (those who did not suffer cognitive impairments) as well as residents who had mild to severe dementia of the Alzheimer's type. But they did not provide separate accommodations for the latter; thus, the living environment was not adapted to the special needs of this population. Neither did they employ caregivers who had special training to take care of such residents. The facility also lacked any special programs designed specifically for Alzheimer's residents prior to the introduction of the services my staff and I provided through the MHNH program.

All 150 of the residents were comingled in the three units. In many cases, alert and oriented residents shared rooms with severely impaired residents. This in itself caused a great deal of friction and distress, and was grossly unfair to both sets of residents.

Theodora was by no means the only resident who created disturbances and exhibited behaviors that were upsetting to the alert and oriented population of the facility. Mixing populations who have differing needs is always problematic and adversely affects the quality of life for all concerned.

Federal regulations expressly mandate that nursing homes must provide an environment and care that meets the specific psychosocial needs of their residents. Yet such arrangements as prevailed at Sunny Hill fly in the face of these mandates. Perhaps the time has come for Congress to add an amendment to OBRA, the Nursing Home Reform Bill, to forbid such housing arrangement in the future.

When we (MHNH) first arrived at Sunny Hill and initiated a cognitive and sensory stimulation program for dementia residents, the caregivers warned us that Theodora would, undoubtedly, cause interruptions and wreck the program. "You'll see," they taunted. "She'll make your life a living hell. You won't get a word in edgewise."

On the first day of the program, Theodora did, indeed, use our group session as an opportunity to entertain us with song and dance and reminiscences of her night club experiences. However, not one of the residents in the group (there were ten of them) objected to her performances. On the contrary, the group was very appreciative of her efforts. They smiled and clapped hands and swayed in harmony with her act. Alzheimer's patients tend to be very tolerant of others, and most of them love music and entertainment.

Theodora was a most delightful addition to the group. Music, exercise, and reminiscing were central components of all our CSS programs. It was a simple matter to incorporate Theodora's performances into the scheduled activities. Instead of being disruptive, her acts served to keep everyone attentive and focused the moment the program commenced. No one ever said: "I'm tired of listening to the same old songs. Why don't you shut up." No one objected to her dancing either.

As long as her performances were accepted without censure, and she received the applause due her, Theodora did not interrupt when we moved on to other segments of the program. During reminiscing, she listened patiently to her peers and waited until it was her turn to share her memories with the group.

She did continue to annoy others in the facility with her performances. And predictably, she reaped the scorn of those residents who found her to be a nuisance.

It made me sad to know how happy and content she could be all day, every day, if she were living in a facility which exclusively served Alzheimer's residents, where no one would object to her entertainment. I wished I could whisk her off to Magnolia Manor.

---

1. Code of Federal Regulations Title 42, Requirements for Long Term Care Facilities, Sec. 483.15 Quality of Life, (a).

Chapter 13

Wilma was a tall, large-boned woman with broad hips and an imposing personality that tended to be intimidating to her peers. She was unusually agile for someone her age and in an advanced stage of Alzheimer's disease. She could no longer communicate verbally, and to compensate for this loss, she asserted herself by pushing away anyone she perceived as being in her way.

She used to come into the dayroom and head straight for the love seat in front of the window, which she considered to be there for her exclusive use. She had a habit of throwing herself onto the seat even if it meant that she had to push someone else off to make room for herself. In fact, she did not tolerate anyone else being seated there, even though it was designed to seat two people quite comfortably.

Some of her peers had learned to quickly get off the love seat as soon as they saw Wilma coming. Those who could not remember the rough treatment she meted out to anyone who displeased her suffered the consequences.

Once seated, Wilma lifted both of her legs, bent at the knees, and rotated her body in one swift motion, until her head was hanging off the front of the seat, and her legs were draped over the back rest. She remained in this upside-down position until one of the caregivers was able to persuade her to either sit up properly or to get off the love seat altogether.

The most effective and ultimately the only way this could be accomplished was to bribe her with a couple of cookies or a cup of chocolate milk. In time, everything that required Wilma's consent and cooperation (getting dressed, brushing her teeth, going to the dining room for meals, etc.) had to be negotiated with her.

According to her husband, Wilma had been a gentle soft-spoken wife and mother who was admired and loved by everyone who knew her. Prior to her descent into AD, she had been very active in community affairs. She had served as president of the Volunteer Services of her hometown, and she had spent many hours each week working in the food pantry helping to provide Meals-on-Wheels for the elderly and disabled. She organized fund-raising events for various charities and worked tirelessly for their success.

"She was the kind of person whose home and heart were always open to anyone who needed a helping hand or a shoulder to cry on," her husband, Gary, said. "She was the most patient and kind person I ever knew." He was still in shock over the changes in Wilma's personality and behavior, which had occurred gradually over a period of six years.

Wilma's husband and children had taken turns caring for her at home during the first several years after she was diagnosed with Alzheimer's. But as the disease progressed, Wilma's behavior became increasingly more difficult to cope with. On the advice of the family physician, they reluctantly placed her into the nursing home.

The first time I encountered Wilma, I was walking along the main corridor of the AD Unit with Enid, one of our clients. Wilma was coming toward us from the opposite direction. As soon as Enid spotted her, she took me by the arm and pulled me over, close to the wall, to give Wilma ample room to pass by us.

"Watch out for this one," Enid confided to me in a whisper, "She's mean—she hits people," and she showed me a fading bruise on her arm where Wilma had punched her.

A week later, Wilma caused more serious injury to another of her peers. Meredith, a new resident, was seated on the love seat when Wilma came along and gestured for her to get off the seat.

Meredith, who was unaware of Wilma's methods of claiming her seat, refused to move, whereupon Wilma unceremoniously took hold of her arms, picked her up off the seat, and dropped her to the floor. Unfortunately, Meredith hit her head on the leg of the table and sustained a bleeding laceration on her forehead, as well as a black eye.

Meredith was rushed to the hospital emergency room for treatment and x-rays. Wilma was transferred to the psychiatric ward of the same hospital. Fortunately, Meredith's injuries proved to be superficial, and her x-rays were negative. But the emotional trauma she had suffered was considerable.

The staff spent extra time with her, as did our MHNH counselor, to comfort and reassure her. Mercifully, due to her short-term memory loss, she quickly forgot the entire incident. Until her laceration healed and the bruising around her eye faded, whenever she glimpsed her face in her bathroom mirror, she commented to her aide, "I wonder how I got so black and blue." But at the same time, whenever she came into the dayroom, she kept her distance from the love seat and chose to sit in a chair at the opposite side of the room, as if she sensed that there was something dangerous about that piece of furniture.

Wilma remained at the psychiatric ward for several weeks. She was put on anti-psychotic medication and kept under observation until her mood and behavior stabilized. When the psychiatric treatment team judged that she no longer posed a threat to the welfare of others, or to herself, she was returned to the nursing home.

For the next several months, Wilma remained stable, and neither her peers nor anyone else had anything to fear from her. She was now as gentle as her husband described her to have been prior to her illness.

Then, as so often happens in such cases, the dosage of her psychiatric medication was reduced and, a few weeks later, reduced again. After several more weeks, since she was still doing well, she was taken off medication entirely.

Predictably, within a short period of time, she began to exhibit signs of acute restlessness and irritability. She began to have difficulty falling asleep at night, and a medication was prescribed for insomnia. This worked to help her fall asleep at bedtime, but by two o'clock in the morning she was again wide-awake and pacing the hall in her pajamas.

Before long, she suffered a full-blown psychotic episode in which she again assaulted one of her peers. This time the injuries she inflicted were more serious. The victim was Natalie, a fragile eighty-five-year-old resident who inadvertently got into Wilma's way. Natalie was walking down the hall when she accidentally bumped into Wilma, who was pacing up and down the hall at the time.

Wilma became so enraged, she picked Natalie up like a rag doll and hurled her against the wall. When Natalie hit the floor, she fractured her wrist, and as she lay screaming in pain, Wilma kicked her viciously in the ribcage before caregivers managed to come to the rescue. The entire incident seemed to have happened in a split second. One of the CNAs had witnessed the assault from the far end of the corridor. She had raced to the scene the moment Wilma had reached out to pick Natalie up, but by the time she arrived at her side it was too late to prevent the deed.

This time, after Wilma was again transferred to the psychiatric ward, she did not return to the nursing home but was placed in a facility for the mentally ill.

One might well ask why Wilma's prescription for psychotropic medication had been discontinued when it was obvious, given her recent history of mental instability, that she needed it. The problem has its roots in past history of how nursing homes dealt with behavior problems in their residents.

Years ago, before OBRA (the Nursing Home Reform Bill) was signed into law, many nursing homes routinely medicated residents who exhibited problem behaviors with tranquilizers and other mind-altering medications in order to render them more manageable. The difficulty was that in addition to reducing or eliminating undesirable behaviors, these drugs also caused the residents to become passive and stuporous. There was ample evidence that many residents were overmedicated and/or inappropriately medicated by the often-indiscriminate use of such drugs.

OBRA has mandated that mind-altering medications, as well as physical restraints, be used only as a last resort. It demands that nursing homes first try other methods of controlling behaviors, such as behavior management protocols, and offering their residents a variety of activities and exercises daily, encouraging them to engage in purposeful activities they enjoy, as a means of reducing discontentment and inappropriate behaviors. These strategies work well for the majority of residents, but not for those who are in a state of psychosis.

If mind-altering drugs are prescribed for a nursing home resident, the physician and the facility staff are required to monitor the resident closely and to document his condition continuously. In addition, the physician is expected to reduce and then discontinue such medications as soon as it appears that the patient is sufficiently improved.[1] The amount of documentation required for each resident who is receiving mind-altering medication is extensive and time-consuming, especially given the fact that many facilities have the minimum staff required by law.

Noncompliance or insufficient compliance can result in censure from the State Health and Human Services Department for both the physician and the facility, unless these protocols are strictly adhered to. The result has been that facilities and physicians have gone to the other extreme and quite commonly reduce or discontinue psychotropic medications as soon as a resident's mood and behavior appear to have stabilized, sometimes with the kind of disastrous result as occurred with Wilma.

It was unfortunate, not to mention unwise, that Wilma's medication was discontinued when it was obvious that she needed it, in addition to regular and timely monitoring by her appointed psychiatrist. There is no doubt that if she had been maintained on an appropriate dosage of her medication, she could, most likely, have remained at the Palm Court without risk of further assaults on others.

The same stringent protocols prevail in the treatment of acute chronic pain. According to federal guidelines it is recommended that facilities first treat a patient's pain with OTC (over-the-counter) medications before resorting to the use of stronger prescription drugs, such as narcotic analgesics. Unfortunately, as a result, many residents with chronic conditions suffer acute pain because they are not receiving sufficiently effective medication.

To this day I am outraged when I think of Elena, a resident who suffered from a severe case of rheumatoid arthritis and was confined to a wheelchair. The intensity of pain she experienced varied from day to day, sometimes from hour to hour. Her physician had prescribed a standing order of Tylenol, once in the morning, and once in the evening, before bedtime.

The first time I saw Elena, she sat hunched over in her wheelchair in front of the counter at the nurses' station. She was crying and begging for medication, her whole face was contorted as the tears rolled down her cheeks.

For several minutes the two nurses behind the counter ignored her. Finally one turned her attention to this distraught resident and admonished her firmly, "Elena, I have already told you I cannot give you any more medication until bedtime. Why don't you go down to the activity program now? You will feel much better if you keep busy with one of your projects instead of dwelling so much on your pain."

Since I had just started to work at this facility, I introduced myself to Elena and offered to wheel her to the activity room where the morning's crafts program was about to begin. She did agree to join the group, but for the entire hour, she continued to sit hunched over in her chair, and it was obvious to everyone that she was in acute pain.

After the program concluded, I took Elena back to her room and stopped at the nurses' station to tell the staff that Elena really appeared to be in great pain. I asked the nurses why she could not have any additional medication. The same nurse who had refused Elena's request earlier told me, "Look, Elena is a chronic complainer. We are used to her tearful performances. You'll get used to them too. It's best to ignore her when she carries on like that."

I was not in the least convinced that Elena was faking pain, and as I got to know her better, I realized the extent to which the staff at this facility was turning a blind eye to her suffering.

Elena had good days, when her pain was bearable, and on those days she was cheerful and enjoyed participating in all the recreation programs. Her room was filled with the evidence of her love of crafts. The needlepoint pillows on her bed, the embroidered wall hangings on her walls, and the beautifully executed small decorative items all testified to the hours she devoted to their creation. She was the life of the party at social events, and she had many friends and several male admirers among her peers.

Unfortunately, she had fewer good days than bad ones, when her pain was so severe that it overwhelmed her and she was unable to do anything but sit hunched over in her wheelchair and moan and cry. On those days she was often rude and had unkind words for her friends. It was obvious to anyone that she needed more and stronger pain medication than she was getting.

Clearly, federal regulations governing the dispensation of psycho-tropic and narcotic pain medications are too rigid. I am not advocating that we go back to the old days, when medications were indiscriminately prescribed without proper monitoring of the patients. But the extensive documentation required for each resident taking such medications needs to be reduced to a more reasonable level. Caregivers simply don't have the time to comply with it as presently required. As a result some residents who would benefit from such medications either don't get them at all, and those who do, often have their medications reduced or withdrawn before it is advisable. Inadequate pain management has been a long-standing serious problem in many of the nation's nursing homes. Some modification in the federal regulations could help to diminish the suffering of residents like Wilma and Elena.

1. Code of Federal Regulations Title 42, Requirements for Long Term Care Facilities, Sec. 483.25, Quality of Care, (2), (i), (ii), (m), (l).

Chapter 14

The first time I entered Marie's room, she was propped up to a sitting position in her bed, and Becky, her aide, was feeding her lunch. It took a long time to complete this task. Marie had to be cued to open her mouth, and cued again to swallow the tiny amounts of pureed food that Becky placed in her mouth with a teaspoon. After every third spoonful of food, Becky picked up a cup of milk from the tray table besides her and held it while she positioned the drinking straw between Marie's lips, and cued her to take a few sips.

Throughout the meal, Becky exhibited great patience and tenderness for Marie. She talked to her sweetly, gently coaxing her, stroking her hand and her cheek now and then to keep her alert. Rarely had I seen such loving devotion delivered along with the nourishment to a nursing home resident.

Marie had been recommended for participation in the MHNH program and, as she was confined to bed, was to receive one-to-one sensory stimulation in her room. Her first session had been scheduled for one o'clock, but I made the decision to reschedule it for a later hour, as it was obvious that Becky needed more time to get Marie cleaned up and settled after the meal. It was also obvious that Marie was exhausted and needed a nap.

Marie had been a resident at the Pine Grove Nursing Home

for eight years. Although she had suffered significant cognitive impairment, prior to her admission, she had been in good physical health. She had been a fun-loving gregarious person who adjusted easily to her new environment. She had enjoyed attending the daily recreation programs. But above all she loved music. She played the piano and she loved to dance.

"You should have seen her when she first came here," Becky, her longtime aide, told me. "She could kick up her heels like nobody else. What a personality. Everybody who came to know her loved Marie."

For the first several years of her stay at Pine Grove, Marie's condition remained relatively stable. After that time her health began to deteriorate rapidly. By the time the MHNH program had been introduced at this facility, she had been confined to bed for three years. All her needs had to be anticipated and met by staff. According to her medical chart, Marie had no living relatives or friends, and her sole contact was with her caregivers.

Despite her severe impairments and her inability to communicate verbally, Marie was able to express a surprising range of feelings by means of grunting, moaning, and a variety of other vocal expressions. It was by no means easy for me to pick up what were often subtle differences in the sounds she produced. It took many sessions with her before I could interpret any significant emotions from these sounds, especially since there was little else by which one could determine what she was feeling.

Marie's facial expression was essentially immobile—what, in mental health jargon, is called presenting a flat affect (an absence of emotions). She could not smile, but she could, on occasion, frown—although it was never clear to me whether her frowns were triggered by involuntary reflexive movement of the facial muscles, or whether they signified feelings of distress or dislike resulting from a specific stimulus.

Though she could not lift her hands or her arms (all her limbs were severely contracted and there was almost no range of motion), she was able to move the fingers of her left hand. When I gently squeezed her hand and asked her to squeeze back, after many trials, she did, if ever so lightly.

Like most Alzheimer's patients in an advances stage of the disease, Marie also had peripheral-vision damage and downward restricted gaze. She could not move the position of her head; thus, her field of vision was confined to a small radius. She could still see objects that were brought within her field of vision, although her responses were selective.

For instance, she did not respond at all to the black-and-white photo portraits (one of Marie as a young girl and one of her parents) that I picked up from her bedside table. However, when she was shown large color flash cards, each depicting a single object (such as a flower or a fruit), Marie seemed to find something familiar in most of these images. She remained attentively focused, and her grunts changed to softer, more pleasant sounds. Of course, I could never be certain whether she recognized and responded to the objects or merely to the bright colors of the images.

Tactile and auditory stimuli proved to be more successful than visual ones, and they triggered more intense responses. I took the splint off her hands that had been placed there to reduce further contraction of her fingers. When I applied hand lotion and massaged her fingers, one by one, and then her hands and arms, Marie closed her eyes and produced a kind of satisfied murmur throughout the procedure indicating that these ministrations pleased her.

When I placed the life-size baby doll on her chest, with the doll's head nestled between Marie's head and shoulder, she closed her eyes again, and soft cooing sounds issued from her throat. She clearly loved the weight of the doll on her chest, as did many of her peers, several of whom had commented, "It feels just like holding a real baby."

I brought in several tapes of different kinds of music to determine if Marie had a preference. One of the tapes was of opera arias sung by Placido Domingo, one was of jazz, and one was of Glenn Miller and his band playing the swing music of the 1940s.

When Marie heard the beginning of the opera tape, her grunts became loud and harsh, signaling her displeasure. The jazz elicited a somewhat milder response but definitely not one of approval.

Her reaction to the swing music, on the other hand, was dramatic and wonderful. Within the first few beats of the music, Marie's eyebrows rose (something I had never seen her do before), and her mouth stretched wide, just for an instant, as if she were attempting to smile. She had stopped grunting and switched to a deep hum. (I had never heard her hum before either). There was no doubt that this was Marie's kind of music, and I played this tape for her every time I came to see her thereafter.

Moments like these, when I had succeeded in finding something that resonated with a severely impaired person, as swing music did with Marie, were very exciting. But they usually were preceded by much trial and error.

Each and every Alzheimer's resident I worked with over the years—and there were so many of them—was unique and responded in his or her own individual manner to the variety of methods and props we employed in providing cognitive and sensory stimulation. During the many months I worked with Marie, I got to know her very well and was able to discern, mostly from the sounds her voice produced, what pleased her and what did not. I was also able to tell when she was tired or did not feel well.

Grunting was a constant feature of Marie's behavior whenever she was awake. She grunted even while Becky was feeding her or while she was being washed and changed. The staff of the unit was accustomed to hearing her voice whenever they passed her room.

In every facility where I have worked there have been one or more residents who grunted or moaned or hummed, more or less continuously. In some cases such repetitive vocal expressions can be a side effect of certain psychotropic medications. However, it can also be triggered by the brain for a variety of other reasons. The psychiatric term for the phenomenon of repetitive vocalizing is *echolalia*. Marie was not on psychotropic medication, but in addition to the brain damage she had suffered due to AD, she had also had a stroke.

One day, when I arrived at the East Wing for my session with Marie, I was informed that she had been transferred the day before to a room on the North Wing. When I entered her room on that wing, I found Marie in a state of disarray and agitation. She was grunting loudly in an angry tone, and the fingers of her left hand—the only part of her body she could move—were picking at the sheet that partially covered her.

I noticed that her hair had not been brushed. Bits of food were caked at the corners of her mouth and also spotted her nightgown as well as the sheet. The odor emanating from her testified to the fact that she needed to be cleaned up and changed. Between grunts, Marie licked her lips, which were dry and cracked. It was apparent that no one had tended to her needs for some time. The evidence suggested that she had been left alone since she had been given her breakfast. Her breakfast tray was still sitting on the tray table beside her bed.

In the bathroom adjoining Marie's room, I soaked a paper towel and grabbed several dry ones as well. I washed her face and dried it. That was all my agency and the facility allowed me to do. I told her I would get someone to take care of her. Then I left her room and went in search of a nurse or an aide, anyone who could alert the person in charge of Marie's care for that day that she was in dire need of attention.

It was just past eleven in the morning, and everyone I saw appeared to be busy getting their residents ready for lunch. I was informed that Marie's aide was on her break and would be back in ten minutes. No one else had either the time or the inclination to tend to her.

There were two nurses behind the desk at the nurses' station engaged in conversation. They were not impressed when I told them that Marie appeared to be uncomfortable and was in need of attention. One of the nurses shrugged her shoulder, "There's nothing we can do. There is no one available to clean her up until her aide comes back from her break." With that, she turned her back on me and resumed her conversation with her colleague.

I asked for permission to give Marie some water to drink, as her dry cracked lips were a sign that she was dehydrated. Permission was granted, and I returned to Marie's room to make her as comfortable as I could while we waited for her aide.

Years ago, nurses took a much more active role in caregiving. These days they leave most of the hands-on caregiving to the nursing assistants. RNs and even LPNs spend most of their time keeping up with the never-ending mountain of documentation required by federal and state requirements for nursing home residents. Most of the remainder of the RN's time is consumed with scheduling assignments for staff, attending staff meetings and care-plan meetings, giving out medication, conferring with physicians, pharmacists, social workers, occupational and physical therapists and other support staff, and dealing with emergencies. Little time remains to actually be spent with the residents.

However, it has been my experience, even today, that truly caring nurses will find the time to take a resident to the bathroom, or to change a diaper when the assigned aide is not available to attend to these tasks in a timely manner. In this case, Marie had already been waiting for a very long time, longer than could be judged reasonable by anyone's standards.

A few days later I was passing by Marie's room on my way to see another client, when I heard her moaning. To me it sounded like a signal of distress.

I went into her room. Her eyes were closed and she did not open them or respond in any other way when I called her name. She continued to moan loudly, as I began to stroke her cheek and massaged her arms. I was sure that Marie was in pain.

I went to the nursing supervisor and informed her of my observation. The supervisor came to Marie's room with me, listened to her moaning for a moment, and declared, "I don't hear anything different. She always sounds like that."

I pointed out that Marie was not responding the way she usually did to stimulation. The supervisor was not impressed. She said, "Frankly, since she was brought to this unit three days ago, I haven't seen any response other than her continuous moans and grunts."

She shouted at Marie several times to open her eyes, and Marie eventually did, but her expression remained fixed and she continued to moan. "You see?" said the supervisor, "She is responding the way she always does. I don't see a problem here."

I explained that I had been working with Marie for several months, and that she was capable of much more than staring into space as she was doing now. I tried once more to convince this nursing supervisor that Marie's moaning indicated to me that she was in distress.

The supervisor called over two of the aides on the wing and asked them, "Do you hear anything different in this resident's moaning from the way she usually sounds?"

After a few seconds of listening to Marie, both girls agreed. "She always sounds like that."

I was convinced that Marie was in pain, and I was becoming really frustrated. "Look," I said, "I may be mistaken, but I feel very strongly that something is wrong with Marie." I pleaded with the supervisor to call Marie's physician and have him examine her.

The supervisor looked at me with contempt. "You are not in charge here," she said. "I would advise you to mind your own business." With that, she turned and walked away.

I knew there was nothing more I could accomplish with the staff on this wing. I suspected that I had probably earned their perpetual hostility, but I was not about to forget about getting Marie the medical attention I believed she needed. The question was how to accomplish this without alienating the entire staff of this wing, possibly of the whole facility and maybe having our contract for mental health services terminated.

I walked over to the East Wing where I knew Becky was on duty until three. I filled her in quickly on my concern for Marie and my encounter with the nursing supervisor. Becky assured me she would go and visit with Marie when her shift was over and said, "If I feel as you do, that Marie needs medical attention, I will talk to the supervisor who comes on duty this afternoon. I have worked with her before. She is much more professional than the supervisor who rebuffed you. I'll let you know what happens."

I was greatly relieved. I thanked Becky and told her she could find me on the North Wing between three and four that afternoon.

Becky was as good as her word. At three-thirty, she came by to tell me that Marie's physician had been called and was expected to come in shortly to examine her.

The following morning when I arrived at the facility, I learned that Marie had been taken to the hospital the previous evening. I found out later that day that she had been operated on for a bowel obstruction. She was doing well and was expected to be returned to Pine Grove within a few days.

I wondered what would have happened if I had not passed by Marie's room the day before and recognized the message of distress in her moaning. Perhaps the staff on the next shift would have picked it up and acted on it—perhaps not.

There is no doubt that it is difficult at times to detect physical illness in an Alzheimer's patient who can no longer verbalize pain or discomfort. Alzheimer's patients exhibit a variety of bizarre behaviors daily, some of which occur without apparent reason, and some of which are repetitive. In Marie's case there had been the additional complication of transfer from one unit to another, just a few days prior to her medical crisis. The staff on the new unit did not know her as well as the staff on her old unit, some of whom, like Becky, had been taking care of Marie for many years.

At the time of her transfer there had been no discernible change in her condition, and her vital signs had been within normal range. The staff had been told that she was a moaner/grunter, and that, in itself, was no cause for concern.

However, the nursing supervisor should have respected the concern of someone who knew Marie well and could differentiate Marie's feelings by the tone of her voice. The supervisor should have acted on my concern by consulting with Marie's physician, instead of being defensive.

Alzheimer's patients are subject to the same variety of diseases and illnesses to which others are vulnerable. Nursing home residents whose mental faculties are intact are usually able to describe any pain or discomfort they are experiencing. In addition, they will, in most cases, complain loudly and persistently, if necessary, until caregivers pay attention and take action to deal with their concerns. Alzheimer's patients are at a great disadvantage in that regard, being completely dependent upon caregivers to anticipate and meet their needs.

Nursing home caregivers need to be especially alert and vigilant with residents who are unable to verbalize, and pick up any clues that could indicate illness. If in doubt, they should err on the side of caution rather than to dismiss clues that a resident may be in need of medical treatment.

*We have to ask ourselves whether medicine is to remain a
humanitarian and respected profession, or a new,
but depersonalized science in the service of prolonged life
rather than diminishing human suffering.*
—Elizabeth Kübler-Ross, MD
On Death and Dying[1]

Chapter 15

Gladys was by far the liveliest member of our cognitive and
sensory stimulation group at the Palm Court Nursing Home's
Alzheimer's unit. Her cheerful disposition contributed much to
the merriment of our daily one-hour sessions. Her sense of humor
and her frequent laughter were so infectious that people were drawn
to her, because the day seemed just a bit brighter for everyone
when Gladys was present.

Yet each morning upon awakening, she had to struggle,
mentally, to make sense of her environment as even the most familiar
routines and aspects of her life became shrouded in mystery
overnight, due to the brain damage that had been caused by
Alzheimer's disease. Some days it took Gladys close to an hour to
reorient herself, and often caregivers had to assist her in this process.

Verbal communication required immense concentration, as key
words she needed to express her thoughts, needs, and wants
frequently eluded her. When her mind failed to yield up the
appropriate words, she often substituted unrelated words that had
similar sounds or letters to the ones she was unable to recall. Once,
while reminiscing about school days, she told the group, "Esther
was my best *fiend* in school."

Sometimes she even made up her own words, quite unaware

that she had done so. Commenting on the quality of the meal she had been served at lunch one day, she said, "This was the most *petricious* meal I ever had."

Her ability to express herself verbally varied from day to day. On some days her memory functioned better than on others. Often, when her problems with word retrieval were most acute, she forgot, midsentence, what she had meant to communicate. She closed her eyes in concentration for a moment, then shook her head, and exclaimed, "Never mind—forget it," and she laughed uproariously. And everyone in the group laughed with her, even though the majority of her peers didn't have the slightest idea what she was laughing about. This ability to laugh when things weren't going right for her was one of the most endearing qualities of Gladys' personality.

One day, she hobbled painfully from her room to the nurses' station and complained that both her big toes were "hurting terribly."

"I never had such a thing happen to me before. I took off my shoes and looked at my toes, but I couldn't see anything wrong with them," she explained.

When the nurse pointed out to her that she had put her shoes on the wrong feet, Gladys looked confused. "What do you mean? How can that be? I only have two feet."

The nurse had to be more specific. "Gladys, you put the right shoe on the left foot and the left shoe on the right foot. That's why your toes are getting pinched. That's why they hurt."

Gladys looked down at her feet. She still didn't seem to understand. The nurse's explanation was too complex for her mind to process. Even the nurse realized that. She pulled up a stool, asked Gladys to be seated, then pulled off her shoes and placed them on the correct feet. "There now, doesn't that feel better?" she asked.

Gladys nodded her head. She finally understood, and she then found the situation so hilarious that she could not stop laughing for several minutes. And everyone present laughed with her. In fact, laughter could be heard, off and on, throughout the unit as one shift told the staff of the next shift about it. There were other incidents that were just as mystifying to Gladys initially, but were just as easily resolved.

Early one morning during the 7:00 AM shift change, the night supervisor of nursing on the South Unit was giving her report to the day shift supervisor just coming on duty. Several of the departing nurses and CNAs were also exchanging information with their counterparts on the dayshift. They were all gathered around the nurses' station when, suddenly, a loud voice could be heard from the other end of the corridor, shouting, "Help! Help! I need help!"

The entire staff turned in the direction of this voice, which was familiar to all of them, and watched as Gladys, once again, came hobbling up to the nurses' station. This time she was not wearing any shoes, and her attire was most unusual, given her usual fastidiousness about how she looked.

She had on a long-sleeved blouse, buttoned to the neck, and a pair of underpants. Her right leg was encased in one pant leg, and Gladys was holding up the pants' waistband with her hands. Her left leg was bare except for a knee sock.

"Look," she told the assembled staff, as she came up to them. "One of my pant legs is gone. Somebody must have cut it off. Who would do such a thing?" She looked positively bewildered.

One look informed the nurses that the second pant leg had been tucked into the first one so neatly that Gladys had not noticed it, and she had inserted her right leg into both pants legs at once.

How this had come about, no one knew for sure, but everyone on staff did know that Gladys liked to fold and put away her own laundered clothes when the laundry workers returned them to her, and often she folded her clothes in ingenious ways.

Once again, everyone including Gladys had a good laugh. It was amazing how she could almost always find humor in the often peculiar situations her failing brain placed her. Most of her peers preferred not to call attention to the puzzling things that happened to them that they could not make sense of, but they would often become so frustrated and angry that they lost control and engaged in inappropriate and sometimes destructive behaviors. Gladys, on the other hand, always came to staff for assistance when she encountered a problem she could not resolve on her own. She took her foibles in stride and did not agonize over them.

Gladys took great care about her appearance. On most days she could still groom and dress herself without assistance or prompting from caregivers. There were other days when it was necessary for staff to lay out her clothes for her, but most of the time she was still able to choose her outfits by herself. All her drawers and her closet had been labeled to tell her where everything was stored.

There were no mirrors in the unit, but Gladys discovered a place where she could look herself over from head to toe, to assure herself that she looked presentable. Every morning, before she sat down for breakfast, she carefully observed herself by looking at her reflection in the glass of the large picture window in the dining room.

This preoccupation with her appearance was rather unusual for someone with advanced Alzheimer's. Most of her peers no longer paid the slightest attention to how they looked. Often they wore clothes inappropriately, in spite of staff's efforts to keep them properly dressed.

The layered look has been popular among Alzheimer's patients long before it came into vogue in the world of fashion. For these patients, dressing themselves becomes a complex and challenging task, and those who still make the attempt to dress themselves often wear several layers of one kind of garment—such as two blouses or shirts, worn one on top of the other, but forgetting to put on a skirt or pants. They also tend to wear clothes inside out or backward. Buttons, snaps, and zippers pose a real problem for them and are, consequently, often ignored.

But Gladys wanted everyone on the unit to look nice and neat, and she was more than willing to help out where help was needed. She went around the unit each day buttoning buttons, pulling up socks, and tucking blouses into skirts or pants. She confined these ministrations to the women on the unit. If one of the men needed adjustment to his clothes, she reported it to the nurses.

There was nothing censorious about these activities; rather she was like a mother hen watching over the welfare of her chicks, making sure they were all taken care of. The staff called Gladys "The Fashion Police," and it was meant affectionately.

There were, however, two residents on the unit of whom Gladys did not approve. These two were Charlie and Harold, who shared a room as well as a penchant for dressing up in women's clothes. Almost daily, Charlie and Harold raided the rooms of female residents and borrowed whatever apparel they could lay their hands on—sweaters, blouses, nightgowns, etc.

It was not unusual to see them parading around the unit, one wearing an embroidered sweater, stretched to the limit over his shirt, the other stuffed into a pink lady's bathrobe. Harold and Charlie just loved to dress up, and the staff, much amused, had dubbed them "The Fashion Plates."

Among the residents, only Gladys appeared to notice that there was something odd about the way these men were dressed. She once walked up to them and addressed herself to Harold, who that day was wearing a flower-patterned cotton housedress.

"Pardon me, mister. Are you a man or a woman?" she asked him.

"Mind your own business," replied Harold, and turned away.

Charlie, who was draped in a fringed turquoise shawl, shook a finger in her face and shouted at her, "Lady, you are no lady!"

Gladys never approached the men again, but every time she saw the pair adorned in female apparel, she muttered, "Those two just don't look right."

Yet she could be sympathetic and accepting of others who exhibited unusual ways of dressing, as for instance Hildie, who insisted on wearing only one shoe, leaving her left foot bare as she wandered around the unit. No matter how many times caregivers hunted down the other shoe and placed it on her bare foot, Hildie would take it off again as soon as their backs were turned. She obviously preferred to walk about with one shoe off, one shoe on, like "My Son John" in the nursery rhyme. Often it was Gladys who retrieved the abandoned shoe and handed it over to a nurse, usually with the admonition, "This lady doesn't like to wear both shoes. Why don't you leave her alone!"

Gladys had three children, two sons and a daughter. Her sons lived in California and traveled east at least once or twice a year to visit their mother in the nursing home. But her daughter, Amy, lived right in town and maintained a close and loving relationship with Gladys, visiting her almost daily.

At least once a week Amy took her mother out to lunch at a restaurant or on a shopping expedition to the nearby mall, but she always brought her back in time to attend the CSS group, which was scheduled for midafternoon, at this facility.

Gladys invariably returned from these outings bubbling with excitement, and eager to tell the group what a wonderful time she had had. Most of the time she had scant recall as to where she had been, but this did not deter her from telling the group in great detail about her outings. She compensated for her short-term memory loss by tapping into her childhood memories to entertain her peers with all sorts of interesting adventures she claimed to have had.

"Amy bought me a candy apple and a hat with a blue feather," she announced to the group one day.

"Where's the hat? Can I see it?" asked Hallie eagerly.

"I put it away in my room. I'll show it to you later," replied Gladys.

"We went to the zoo too," she continued.

"What kind of animals did you see?" Edith wanted to know.

"We saw cats and kittens and dogs and puppies," Gladys told her.

"When I went to the zoo I saw elephants and tigers and lions," declared Max, frowning.

"Well, we saw those too," stated Gladys. She enjoyed having the group's attention.

"Did you eat in a restaurant?" asked George, who was always interested in food.

"Oh yes," said Gladys. "We ate in a place that was way up high on top of a mountain. We had to ride up there in a car that was tied to a string."

"There's no such thing," grumbled George.

"Do you mean a cable car?" I asked Gladys. I knew she had lived in Switzerland for a time when she was a child.

"Yes, I think so. Anyway, we were above the clouds. That's how high up this place was," she continued.

The fact that there were no such high mountains within thousands of miles from where we were went right by the group. Not even George questioned this part of Gladys's confabulation. But everyone wanted to know what she had eaten at this restaurant above the clouds.

"Oh, a little of this, a little of that. It's what we always have," is how Gladys answered this question.

"What does that mean?" asked George, impatiently. 'Did you have chicken or hamburger or pizza, or what?"

"Of course," replied Gladys. "We had that too."

"All of it?" asked George, incredulously.

"Yes, all of it," confirmed Gladys.

"Boy!" exclaimed George, "I wish I could eat in a restaurant like that."

"I'll ask my mother if you can come with us next time," Gladys told him, completely forgetting that it was her daughter, not her mother, who was taking her out to lunch these days.

This was just one of many similarly tall tales that Gladys told the group. She always spoke with such animation and such confidence that it was rare for anyone to question the truthfulness of her stories.

Gladys was much admired by her peers for the entertainment she provided. She contributed much to the high level of attentiveness of the members of this CSS group. Her enthusiastic participation in the program acted as a catalyst on her peers and encouraged them to be less reticent in their participation.

Gladys had been a resident at the Palm Court for close to ten years by the time the MHNH program was initiated at the facility. Her disease had been stabilized at midlevel for six years by the time I met her, and she continued to remain on that plateau, physically, mentally, and emotionally, for the next several years.

The staff was amazed how well Gladys continued to function after so many years with AD. It almost seemed as if the disease process in Gladys had been arrested for good, while it continued to progress in others who had had AD for a much shorter period of time.

The day after Gladys was taken to her daughter's home to celebrate her eighty-fourth birthday with her family, she fell in the dining room and sustained a compound hip fracture. In the hospital she developed complications and nearly died of pneumonia. She did survive that crisis and was able to return to the nursing home after several weeks. Her bones were mending, and, thanks to the dedicated physical therapist at the Palm Court, she even learned to walk again. After several months she graduated from her wheelchair to a walker and then to a cane.

But she remained physically frail and her appetite was poor. She never quite regained her strength, and the vitality which had been a hallmark of her personality prior to her accident had vanished. All of a sudden, she seemed to deteriorate rapidly, and simultaneously, on all fronts.

Gladys had come back from the hospital completely confused and disoriented. She didn't recognize any of her caregivers or her roommate. Her physician felt this was, at least in part, due to the combined trauma of the accident, the displacement from her familiar environment to the hospital, and the pain medication she had been receiving. He believed that over time, this confusion would diminish. The occupational therapist worked with Gladys to encourage her to resume her independent dressing and grooming, but Gladys no longer cared about her appearance. She would look at a blouse or a pair of pants and couldn't figure out how to put them on. Instead of brushing her teeth, the staff found her using her toothbrush to comb her hair. Her language skills had become reduced to the use of single random words. She began to have difficulty understanding even the simplest verbal communication. She had acute episodes of anxiety. She became very restless and took to pacing the hallways in a typical "sundowning" pattern (continuous pacing by Alzheimer's patients, especially toward the end of the day). She was still using a cane and her balance was precarious. Caregivers and her physician decided to place her back into a wheelchair, to eliminate the risk of further falls and injuries.

When her daughter came to visit her, Gladys no longer seemed to recognize Amy as her daughter, but called her "Mamma." The first time she did so, her daughter visibly froze for a moment, and then fled. Watching her mother deteriorate so drastically was unbearably painful for Amy. Her response was to withdraw from her mother physically, as well as emotionally. Her visits became less frequent and, eventually, dwindled to one short visit on the weekends.

It was noted by staff that Amy no longer hugged or kissed her mother. In fact, she never touched her at all anymore. During her short visits, she remained seated across from Gladys, at a distance, and her communication was stiff and formal, even as Gladys reached out to her, with both arms, babbling incoherently, and obviously seeking some affection, some reassurance from this woman whom she now thought of as her mother. But Amy was unable to bridge the void that existed between them, and it was caregivers who comforted Gladys after her daughter left.

Since Gladys was no longer the lively, cheerful person her peers had known, they too withdrew and ignored her. But she was so needy of attention that she grabbed and held on to anyone who came near her. Sometimes she babbled and her voice became louder and louder, often ending in piercing shrieks until someone, usually a caregiver, paid attention to her.

She responded well to a gentle back rub; it seemed to calm her. And if one reached out and offered her a hand, she would hold it tenderly in hers and stroke it with her other hand for a moment, and then she would look up with such gratitude in her eyes, it could melt a stone. Those of us who had such moments with her always felt guilty that there wasn't more we could do for her, that we didn't have more time to spend with her.

But there were also times when she sat quietly in her wheelchair staring into space for long periods of time, having withdrawn her attention, and it appeared that she had no awareness of her environment. Some of the staff ignored her when she was in this state, and one caregiver commented to me, "I'm glad when she withdraws like that. Lately, it's the only time when she doesn't cause a scene and pull at you." But other caregivers continued to make an effort to pull Gladys out of this trancelike state and to interact with her.

Gladys had to be fed by staff now, as her motor skills had also declined and she could no longer hold the utensils to feed herself, nor could she maintain the concentration needed to eat her food. Sometimes she fell asleep in the midst of being fed. It was particularly important during meals to keep her as alert as possible. Her appetite had been diminishing for some time, and she was losing weight.

She had developed difficulty swallowing. There was concern that her choking episodes could result in aspirating food particles into her lungs. All her meals had to be pureed and liquids thickened to prevent choking due to her weakening swallowing reflexes. She was given smaller but more frequent meals.

She had other problems as well. She suffered recurring urinary tract infections and was also being treated for edema. Clearly, she was losing ground in spite of the efforts of the treatment team to attend to all her medical problems and to get an adequate amount of nutrition into her system. "She is skin and bones" was how one of her CNAs described her.

At this juncture, her physician met with the nursing home care team and Gladys's family. One of her sons flew in from California to participate in the consultation. The physician recommended a PEG tube (percutaneous endoscopic gastrostomy) for Gladys. This tube would be inserted directly into her stomach through the stomach wall, and thereafter she would receive all her nutrition in liquid form through this tube rather than by mouth. "That way we can be sure that she will get adequate nutrition and the risk of choking will be eliminated," explained the physician.

In light of their mother's frail condition, Gladys's children were reluctant to consider such a drastic invasive procedure. But the physician then told them bluntly that without the stomach tube their mother would die of starvation. This was so unacceptable to Gladys's children that they decided to go ahead with the procedure immediately.

Afterward, Gladys developed a skin infection at the surgical site that did not improve despite the antibiotics being pumped into her system and the topical treatment of the wound. Neither did she regain any of the weight she had lost in recent weeks. On the contrary, she continued to lose weight. In addition, she now suffered from congestive heart failure and was put on oxygen to ease her labored breathing.

She experienced much pain and discomfort, which was apparent from her moans and groans and her effort to pull out the tube and tear away the dressing around it. Her hands were placed in padded mittens to prevent her from pulling at the tube. Her family hired private-duty nurses who took over every aspect of her care around the clock. They monitored her continuously and kept her as comfortable as possible.

Gladys's skin was now so fragile that she developed bedsores. Her heels and her elbows in particular were so sore that they bled. A lambskin pad was placed beneath her body. Her elbows were pillowed in down cushions, and her heels were covered with padded booties. The room was kept at a temperature that permitted her to be covered with the lightest of bedsheets so as to avoid pressure on any part of her body.

Gladys had little conscious awareness of her caregivers or her surroundings now. Despite all the care and attention she received, she died less than three weeks after the insertion of the PEG tube.

What the physician had failed to tell her children was that when the PEG tube was inserted into her stomach, Gladys was already in the final stage of Alzheimer's disease. So the nutrition delivered through the tube into her system could no more prevent her from starving to death than food taken by mouth could have done; because by this point all of her vital bodily systems were breaking down and metabolic processes had ceased to function. Yes, Gladys had been dying of starvation, but she had also been dying of the failure of her kidneys, her liver, her heart, her lungs. She had been dying of Alzheimer's disease.

One has to wonder: Did this physician know that Gladys was in the final stage of AD, that she was, in effect, already dying when he recommended the insertion of a PEG tube?

There are medical conditions for which a stomach tube can save and prolong the life of a patient, sometimes for years. I have personally known and worked with several such patients in the nursing homes, and they were doing well. But when a person has reached the final stage of AD, a stomach tube is useless, because no treatment or medical procedure, currently available, can reverse the process of metabolic breakdown once it has begun, nor can it improve the patient's condition—or hold off death.

It is cruel to subject a person in such a state to any invasive procedure. Gladys could have been kept hydrated by an intravenous drip of appropriate fluids, and other supportive noninvasive measures could have kept her comfortable and free of pain through the final days of her life, letting nature take its course, instead of making her dying so much more of an ordeal both for her and for her family.

After Gladys's death, her daughter, Amy, told the nursing home staff that the family would not have opted to put their mother through this final medical intervention if they had known how grave Gladys's condition was. They would have liked to spare her the additional pain and discomfort in her last days.

Most of the nursing home staff involved in Gladys's care knew that a stomach tube could not improve her condition, but no one had dared to speak up. For better or worse, a physician's judgment and recommendations regarding medical treatment was not to be questioned or contradicted by nursing home staff at any time.

It is difficult to understand Gladys's physician's decision and recommendation to her family. But then, it should by no means be taken for granted that this particular physician understood the dynamics of end-stage Alzheimer's disease. Today there are many physicians who are very knowledgeable about AD and are supportive to patients and their families in dealing with the disease. But there are still physicians taking care of Alzheimer's patients in the nursing homes whose knowledge about AD appears to be less than thorough.

While writing this book, I asked a number of physicians what they had been taught about AD in medical school. Most of them could not recall having been taught anything specific about it except that it is one of the diseases of old age that causes dementia and ultimately results in death.

To be fair, my questions were directed to a very small sampling of fifteen physicians who practice various medical specialties today. All of them had graduated from medical school at least ten or more years ago. Most of them confessed that they did not know much about AD. Only three of the fifteen had kept up with the research that has generated a wealth of new information about the disease and the specific ways it affects its victims.

This should not come as a surprise when one considers that according to the Alzheimer's Association, just twenty years ago AD was not even on the radar screen of most of the medical profession.

---

1. Elizabeth Kübler-Ross, *On Death and Dying* (New York: The Macmillan Company, 1969), 11.

Companionship is food and drink for the human spirit.
—William H. Thomas
Life Worth Living[1]

Chapter 16

All of us who provided mental health services in the nursing homes have at one time or another witnessed caregiving that, although it could not be legally classified as neglect or abuse, at the very least, demonstrated insensitivity and lack of respect for the residents.

Whenever we did observe such behaviors, we brought them to the attention of the offender's supervisor. But no matter how diplomatically we approached them, this was not always appreciated. We were not employees of the nursing homes but rather of the community mental health service provider, and if the nursing homes were dissatisfied with our services or our conduct, they could easily dismiss us by canceling the contract for our services. We had to take care not to overstep the bounds of what the nursing homes deemed appropriate behavior for us.

Our employers provided us with continuous in-service education on a variety of issues pertaining to our work with mental health clients. One of these in-services addressed the subjects of *abuse and neglect*. The lecture was given by a representative of the Florida Health and Rehabilitation Services' (HRS) legal department.

We were informed that unless the body of the alleged victim betrayed visible signs of abuse (cuts, bruises, broken bones, etc.) or neglect (signs of dehydration, emaciation, and/or other medically provable evidence), an incident did not legally constitute abuse or neglect, and the alleged perpetrator would not be prosecuted.

We asked, "What about a resident's emotional distress caused by abuse that does not result in visible signs on the body, such as a resident being pulled or yanked about, or otherwise being treated with disrespect?" We had all witnessed such acts by caregivers, at one time or another.

The legal expert from HRS shrugged and repeated, "It is not considered abuse, legally, unless there is visible evidence of injury. By all means, report any incidents you believe warrant investigation," he continued, "but I can tell you right now that unless there is proof of injury, there won't be any consequences for the alleged offender."

This was not only shocking to us, but it left us feeling upset and frustrated, because we believed that treating any resident with less than consideration, kindness, and respect is abusive and should never be tolerated. Any behaviors that caused a resident emotional distress were unacceptable to us.

Although many of the caregivers were doing a fine job of caring for the residents, there were a few, in every facility we served, who treated them with indifference or rudeness. Such treatment can be just as hurtful as physical injury, and we often witnessed this kind of abuse or heard about it from clients in our sessions with them.

One of our nursing home specialists related the following complaint made by Olivia, one of her clients. This client reported that the nurse who dispensed medication on her unit entered her room every morning without knocking at her door first and, without so much as a greeting, commanded her to open her mouth, whereupon she shoved in a spoonful of medication and then left without another word.

When the counselor asked Olivia why she didn't tell the nurse that her rudeness offends her, she replied, "I tried that, I told her she is supposed to knock before she comes into my room. And I even told her that from now on I wouldn't open my mouth unless she asked me politely. Well, she just left in a huff and reported to her supervisor that I had refused to take my medication."

When asked if she had explained to the supervisor how rude the medication nurse had been, Olivia shook her head, "Oh, I couldn't do that," she said, "if I snitched on her, she'd get even more nasty. Besides, I'm not the only one she treats like that. But none of us are prepared rat on her."

Because this client was seriously upset about the situation, but refused to report it, the counselor made it her business to be present in Olivia's room the following morning when the medication nurse entered. The nurse greeted the counselor, but again ignored the resident except to ask her to open her mouth for her medication. When Olivia refused to confront the nurse about her rudeness, the counselor took it upon herself to speak to the nursing supervisor about the problem.

At the next session, the counselor asked Olivia if there had been any improvement in the nurse's behavior.

"It depends on what you call improvement," she replied. "She knocks on my door now before she comes in, and she says 'please' when she asks me to open my mouth. But she looks at me with such contempt that I feel worse, every time I see her, than I did before. I can tell you, seeing the nasty expression on that girl's face first thing every morning is a hell of a way to have to start the day."

However, it wasn't only nursing department personnel whose behavior sometimes caused the residents distress. One of my own clients, Tanya, who was confined to bed, tearfully confided to me one day that her attending physician routinely came to examine her without ever speaking to her directly or acknowledging her as a person.

"I always say, 'Hello, Dr. Johnson,' every time he comes to see me, but he never says hello to me. He never even looks me in the eye. He only talks to the nurse," she sobbed. "He treats me like I don't exist. It hurts to be so completely ignored."

This particular physician had a reputation for rudeness, not only to his patients, but to everyone with whom he came in contact at the nursing home. One has to wonder why such people choose to work in the healing professions. They do more harm than good, regardless of how skilled they are in their respective specialties.

After several counseling sessions, Tanya mustered the courage to confront her physician about his rudeness, and he apologized ("His face turned red with embarrassment," she reported, gleefully), and thereafter he behaved in a more civilized manner. It did wonders for Tanya's self-esteem.

Neither Olivia nor Tanya suffered from dementia. Both were alert and oriented, and while they had found it difficult to confront those who had failed to exercise even the most rudimentary forms of courtesy, their problems were dealt with because they were able to verbalize and share their distress with their counselors.

On the other hand, those who suffer from Alzheimer's disease or other forms of dementia are rarely able to influence how they are being treated. Unfortunately, there are still caregivers who believe that to communicate and interact with a person who has severe dementia is a waste of time because that person has lost the ability to comprehend and appreciate communication.

A caregiver who refuses to acknowledge a resident, who fails to communicate with him and ignores his right and his need to be included in the community of his peers, has judged him to be unworthy of attention and has condemned him to nonperson status. Such behavior toward a resident is abominable, but it is particularly cruel when perpetrated on a person who is helpless and entirely dependent upon the caregivers.

Whenever and wherever such behavior by a caregiver is observed in a nursing home, it must be reported to the appropriate authority of the facility. And although the offense against a resident may not be legally classified as abuse or neglect, it must be dealt with to assure that it does not happen again. Ultimately, it is the responsibility of the management to protect residents from anyone who violates their rights to be treated with respect and whose behavior cause them distress.

---

1. William H. Thomas, *Life Worth Living: How Someone You Love Can Still Enjoy Life in a Nursing Home—The Eden Alternative in Action* (Acton, MA: VanderWyck & Burnham, 1996), 28.

Frank is so demented, so unresponsive,
that it doesn't matter where he is.

—A Nurse

Chapter 17

At the Pine Grove Nursing Home, our CSS group meeting commenced each weekday morning at ten o'clock in a small sitting room on the South Wing. To reach this location, one had to walk down a long corridor passing by residents' rooms on either side.

I traversed this corridor repeatedly each morning in the process of gathering my Alzheimer's clients from their respective wings (there were three) and bringing them to the sitting room. By 9:50 AM, when I was usually on my last trip, nearly all the rooms on the South Wing were unoccupied, except for those few in which residents were confined to bed.

The Pine Grove staff encouraged the residents to be out of their rooms most of the day as a means to reduce self-isolation. The majority of the residents gathered in the recreation room for the facility's morning program. Of those who chose not to attend, some went to the dayroom to watch TV, play cards, and socialize, while others sat outside on the patio to get some fresh air before it got too hot for comfort.

Walking down the corridor each morning with the last of my group members, I encountered primarily housekeeping staff cleaning rooms, and perhaps a CNA or two bringing wheelchair-bound residents to activities. However, there was one room that was always occupied by a male resident in a wheelchair whenever I passed by his room. I could not see his face as he was always seated with his back to the open door.

The first several days I noticed him, I did not give it much thought, as my staff and I had just recently started to work at this facility, and we were not yet familiar with all the routines of the place, nor with all the residents and staff. But it did strike me as peculiar that this resident was always placed in the same position—with his back to the open door—facing what appeared to be a blank wall. He sat as still as a statue, and I never once saw even a flicker of movement from him whenever I walked past his room.

After several days, my curiosity got the better of me, and I asked one of the nurses why this resident was never brought out of his room.

"You mean Frank?" she asked. "Oh, he is so demented, so unresponsive, that it doesn't matter where he is."

I asked the nurse if it was OK for me to visit him. "I'd like to see if I can elicit some response from him."

The nurse snorted in derision, and said, "Honey, be my guest—and good luck."

I walked into Frank's room and finally got to see him face-to-face. He was a good-looking man; he had a full head of fluffy white hair and bushy eyebrows above large but expressionless hazel eyes. His finely chiseled face was clean shaven but without animation. Both his hands were in splints to prevent his fingers from contracting.

I noticed that his fingernails were clean and well trimmed (the state of a resident's fingernails is one indication of the quality of care a facility provides). It was obvious that Frank was receiving excellent physical care. He was a big man with broad shoulders, and his wheelchair was one of the wider ones that accommodated his bulk comfortably.

He sat very straight and upright in his chair, but as always, he didn't move a muscle; even his eyes barely blinked. I did my best to get his attention, and I managed to make eye contact with him. I called his name and talked to him, but his facial expression remained flat and his eyes dull. He did not acknowledge my presence in any way. As the nurse had said, he was entirely unresponsive. Nevertheless, I just did not feel comfortable about his being left alone in his room all by himself without any stimulation. There were other residents in the facility who exhibited minimal awareness of their environment, but they were brought out of their rooms daily. Although they were unable to participate actively in the communal life of the other residents, they were included. Frank, however, left in his room without human contact most of the day, was treated as a nonperson. It troubled me deeply.

The next day, I approached Ellen, the social service director, and asked her if I might include Frank in the MHNH program. I pointed out to her that since Frank had dementia, he was entitled to receive mental health services.

This request, on my part, was highly irregular. We (MHNHP) did not solicit for clients. As a rule the request for our services on behalf of their residents came from the facilities. Although it was uncertain whether Frank would derive any benefit, I felt that including him in the program was the right thing to do. I had already seen an increase in animation and alertness of several other dementia clients after only a few days of participation.

Ellen agreed with me that we should try Frank in the program, and we both set the wheels in motion to obtain the necessary permissions from Frank's legal guardian and his attending physician. One of my first tasks in the process of assessment and documentation was to acquaint myself with Frank's medical and personal histories. His medical chart provided the following information:

Frank was born in Germany in 1912, an only child, and immigrated to the United States with his parents in 1921 when he was nine years old. The family settled in New Jersey where Frank's uncle Otto, his father's brother, assisted them in obtaining work and housing. Frank completed high school in 1929 and accepted a job as clerk in a local business that manufactured paper products. He worked his way up the ladder in this company and eventually attained the position of district sales manager. He met and married his wife Ingeborg, an immigrant from Sweden, in 1940. According to Frank's guardian, the marriage was a very happy one although the couple remained childless. Frank served in the U.S. Army overseas from 1943 until the end of WWII, when he returned to continue his employment at the paper products company. In 1955, the couple moved to Mexico City where Frank took over the management of a new branch office his firm had established there.

The couple prospered and enjoyed life in Mexico until 1978, when an auto accident resulted in Ingeborg's death, and Frank suffered spinal injuries that left him paralyzed from the waist down.

Unable to continue to work and severely depressed, Frank moved to Florida upon the urging of his friend and attorney, Ralph H., a widower himself, who had invited Frank to share his house in Fort Lauderdale.

The two friends got along well, and slowly Frank began to come to terms with the double tragedy of losing his wife and his mobility. The two men shared many leisure activities such as fishing, playing cards, and attending sports and social events in their community.

Then, in 1984, Frank began to exhibit episodes of serious mood swings. His memory began to fail, and he suffered episodes of confusion and disorientation. Ralph coped as best he could with Frank's failing health over the next two years. At that point Frank was tested by a neurologist and diagnosed with dementia of the Alzheimer's type. Shortly thereafter, Ralph H. was appointed Frank's legal guardian, as the latter had no living relatives. On the advice of Frank's personal physician, Ralph placed him into the Pine Grove Nursing Home, one of the best facilities in the area.

According to Ellen, the SSD, Frank had initially had a difficult period of adjustment. But with the help of medication his mood swings subsided, and he became more relaxed and accepting of life at the facility. Within several weeks, he had made friends with select male peers and became an active participant in the daily recreational programs.

"When he first came here, he spoke both English and Spanish

fluently, although he did have problems with word retrieval in both languages," said Ellen. "Our kitchen staff, most of whom are Mexican immigrants, loved to converse with him in their native language," she continued.

"How long has it been since Frank lost the ability to use language?" I asked.

"It happened very rapidly about a year and a half ago," replied Ellen," and as I recall, he lost both languages almost simultaneously. For a short period of time he was still able to comprehend what was communicated to him in English, but soon even that was lost. After that, he seemed to just shut down. I mean he just stopped responding to any stimuli."

Permission was granted for Frank to join the MHNH program, and every morning I stopped by his room to bring him to the CSS group. He never responded to my cheerful greeting, and one could not even say that he was a passive observer in the group. At first he appeared to be completely oblivious to what was going on around him. But that did not deter me from my continued attempts to interact with him.

One of our daily activities was the ball-tossing exercise for which I employed a large beach ball because it was light in weight and easy to grasp and hold on to. I went around the circle of the group and tossed the ball to each resident in turn, and they threw it back to me. This exercise was an important component of the program. It was an activity that even the most highly impaired residents could participate in.

I frequently resorted to the ball tossing more than once during the program. One of the characteristics of AD is a short attention span. So when I noticed that my group's attention began to wander from whatever activity we were engaged in, I switched to another round of ball tossing. It gave me the opportunity to interact with each participant on a one-to-one basis.

When I had first started the group sessions, some of the residents no longer even remembered what a ball was for, and had no idea what to do with one. I had to teach them, step by step, how to catch the ball and throw it. Naturally, our ball tossing was done at very close range. In some cases I literally dropped the ball into a person's lap, and all they had to do was grasp it and give it a light toss. For some of our residents that was a major accomplishment. Often their throws went far and wide, and they loved it when the ball went past me, and I lunged and lurched about to try and catch it. There was a lot of clowning on my part, and lots of laughter and giggles from the residents during ball tossing. We always did these exercises to lively music, which also contributed to the cheerful mood of the group.

I started to work with Frank the same way I had with other severely impaired residents. When I first held up the ball in his field of vision to get his attention, he exhibited not the slightest sign of interest in the ball or in me. But when I placed the ball in his lap and guided both his hands to touch it and hold it, he looked at it and gripped it more tightly.

I then moved his arms up and down, several times—just a little—to bounce the ball on his lap. Afterward, it was difficult to pry the ball out of his hands, because he could not let it go. He didn't know how. However, I was so encouraged by our small success that after the group session was over, I worked some more with Frank, repeating the motions with the ball.

After several days, Frank began to anticipate the ball when I stepped up to him with it, and he paid attention. After several more days of repeating the same exercise, I actually tossed the ball in his lap and watched in amazement as he placed his hands around it, spontaneously, and gripped it tightly without any intervention from me. He held the ball in his lap and began to hum. It was a monotonous hum that appeared to come from deep within him. He continued to hum as I guided his hands through the motion of bouncing the ball.

Step by step, day by day, and very slowly, Frank relearned to catch the ball at close range, and hold on to it. His humming became part of the exercise, and in fact, he began to hum as soon as he took note of the ball.

Then one day, after we had practiced the motion of bouncing the ball, he actually lifted it in his hands a few inches off his lap, opened his fingers to release it, and watched it roll out of his hands and hit the floor, where it bounced several times before it rolled away. Frank's humming became deeper and louder and appeared to me to be resonating with a sense of satisfaction.

It took some time, weeks, in fact, but eventually Frank was able to catch the ball and toss it back to me. It took great effort and immense concentration for him to accomplish this feat. The range of motion in his arms was limited. It was difficult for him to grasp the ball with his splinted hands. His whole body shook with the energy he expended in the forward motion required to give the ball momentum and to release the grip of his hands upon it, to let it go.

The staff of the facility, some of whom had observed my work with Frank, initially expressed contempt and disbelief that I would waste my time to teach Frank something that they believed to be beyond his abilities. But as the weeks went by, and they could see some progress, they apologized and acknowledged that maybe there was some merit in my efforts.

Frank continued to pay little attention to any of the other activities of the group. He could not participate in the cognitive stimulation exercises, but he appeared to enjoy the ball-tossing exercises. At least it seemed so to me, based on the fact that he exhibited increasing animation during these interactions.

Several months later, Ellen, the SSD, approached me after one of our group sessions and informed me that she had just spoken to Frank's guardian, Ralph H., who called her from time to time to inquire about his welfare. She said that she told him about my work with Frank.

"He was very pleased," Ellen said, "and he would like to talk to you about it." She handed me a note with his phone number.

When I called him later that afternoon, Mr. H. told me how surprised he was to hear that Frank had shown some improvement. I cautioned him that Frank's responses to my efforts with him could not be classified as improvement, that rather his recent accomplishments meant that he had some residual abilities which, unfortunately, no one had been aware of, and consequently no one had made any attempt to encourage him to use them.

Mr. H. wanted to know how I had discovered these residual abilities and been able to get Frank to use them. I filled him in on the details, and he expressed the hope that with my continued efforts Frank might improve, and perhaps, even be able to regain his understanding and use of language. "You know, he always was a very intelligent man."

I regretfully disabused him of this hope and gave him a more realistic view of Alzheimer's disease. Before we ended the conversation, Mr. H. said, "Ursula, that's a German name, isn't it?" And I assume by your accent that you were born in the old country?"

I confirmed that I had indeed been born and raised there.

"Did you ever talk to Frank in German?" he asked. "You know, he continued to speak his native language well. He frequently traveled to Germany after the war, and he was a member of a German Singing Club in New York that sang German folk songs at various community events."

Mr. H. further told me that Frank had been christened *Franz*, but had changed his name to Frank when he became a U.S. citizen.

This was interesting information. I knew that when Alzheimer's patients begin to lose the ability to use language, they generally forget any languages they had learned subsequent to the first language learned in infancy. And they generally revert back to this language before, ultimately, all language skills are lost. I wondered if Frank might have retained any familiarity with his native language.

The next morning when I picked Frank up at his room to take him to group, I greeted him in German and used his German name: "*Guten Morgen, Franz. Wie geht es ihnen?*" (Good morning, Franz. How are you?)

Frank nodded his head vigorously, and began to hum. At the same time a smile appeared on his face. It was the first time I had ever seen him smile.

I repeated the question, "Wie geht es ihnen, Franz?" The humming continued and grew louder.

I had the distinct impression that the language sounded familiar to him and that he recognized his given name. But it occurred to me, at the same time, that I might be mistaken, that his response— such as it was—related only to the attention I was giving him. He kept on humming, but his smile had already faded away. I wanted to see that smile back on his face.

I knelt down in front of his wheelchair, took both of his hands in mine, and said, *"Franz, geht es ihnen gut?"* (Are you well?) His finger tightened on my hands so hard it was painful.

"Gut, gut," he said, as he pumped my hands up and down.

I was astonished. The most I had hoped for was that perhaps the language might sound familiar, and that he might possibly understand a few words and let me know if he did by means of nonverbal communication, such as nodding his head, and humming. After all, according to caregivers, he had not uttered a word in any language for more than a year.

I regretted that I had to terminate our interaction at this point, but it was time to start the group session. The participants had already been assembled in the sitting room, and I did not wish to keep them waiting.

During our one-to-one ball-tossing exercise, I did speak to him in German and called him Franz instead of Frank, but there was no further verbalization from him, and he seemed oddly distracted.

The following morning I went to his room early so that we would have a full fifteen minutes together before group. He responded as he had the previous day to my greeting in German by humming and smiling, briefly. Again he answered, *"Gut, gut,"* to my question if he was well, but only after I myself had used the word *gut* several times.

I had come armed with a set of large flash cards depicting simple everyday objects such as a house, a car, and various common fruits and vegetables. Holding up a card and pointing to it to focus his attention, I called out the German name of the object shown and waited a few seconds, then asked him, "*Was ist das?*"

Frank looked at the picture blankly but began to hum again. I went through the routine with five different cards and got no response except the continued humming.

The next card pictured an apple. As I held it up, a new thought occurred to me, namely that the objects in pictures might be too abstract for Frank. Perhaps he could not read the pictures. I remembered that I had brought an apple with my lunch that day.

After group, I took the apple to Frank, held it out to him, and said: "*Das ist ein Apfel.*" Frank looked at it for a moment, then repeated the word "*Apfel*" loud and clear. I then asked him in German if he liked apples, and he replied, "*Gut, gut,*" nodding his head affirmatively.

Clearly, this response called for a reward. I went to the nurses' station and asked for permission to give Frank the apple. Then I took my apple to the kitchen and asked the aide to peel it and cut it up into small thin pieces for Frank.

Frank enjoyed eating the apple. However, I could not tell if he connected the pieces of apple with the whole apple I had shown him earlier, but that did not matter. What mattered was that he had come alive in a way that no one thought him capable anymore. What mattered was that he no longer spent his days seated in his room facing a blank wall.

I continued to work with Frank in our cognitive and sensory stimulation group and also in one-to-one sessions. Initially I had hopes of triggering lost memories, reawakening and reactivating lost abilities.

But soon I came to realize that my expectations were unrealistic, and I came to accept that *gut* was the only word Frank could say and know the meaning of. *Gut* is a good word, especially if one can say only one word. It is an affirmative word, a positive word that is useful in many different contexts, but all related to a sense of approval and satisfaction. How do you feel? Are you comfortable? Do you like your dinner? Would you like to play ball? And Frank used the word to answer all these questions and more. He not only used the word *gut* to convey satisfaction when something pleased him, but to say "Thank you" as well.

Of course, I also attempted to elicit some response to the English language, but there I hit a blank wall. Frank only looked bewildered or frowned, as if the sound jarred his sensibilities. Other times he simply ignored the speaker. He definitely seemed to prefer the sound of his mother tongue.

Perhaps if someone could have spent more time with Frank daily, consistently, at an earlier stage of his illness, he might have retained verbal abilities for a longer time. There is some truth in the adage, "use it or lose it."

Unfortunately, there had been no CSS programs for dementia residents at this facility prior to the implementation of the mental health program. Residents like Frank, who had no regular visits from family and friends received relatively little stimulation. Despite his inability to use language, Frank, like so many other residents was not incapable of appreciating attention from others. He retained the need for human contact and for stimulation that we all share, even though he was no longer able to communicate this to his caregivers.

During the years I worked with Alzheimer's patients in the nursing homes I had many memorable encounters with severely impaired residents, but perhaps the most memorable was spent one morning with Frank.

I had recently discarded my old hi-fi player in favor of an audio tape player, so I decided to donate my now-obsolete LPs to Pine Grove, which used a record player in the little sitting room. Among my old records was one of German folk songs sung by a male choir.

After group the following day, I kept Frank seated in the room to play this special record for him. I was curious whether he would recognize any of the songs. My back was turned to him while I placed the LP on the turntable and adjusted the volume.

As the voices of the choir filled the room with the first

sentimental song "*Sah ein Knab ein Röslein stehn*" I turned around and could hardly believe my eyes. Tears were streaming down Frank's face. When I walked up to him, he grabbed both my hands in his and pulled them to his chest where he held them in a vice-like grip, and said, "*Gut, gut.*"

He was trembling with emotion, and for a moment I felt that perhaps this was too much for him. I was deeply moved myself by Frank's reaction. With each subsequent song Frank's eyes flooded anew and he nodded his head in recognition. I was glad when the recording ended and he could recover his emotional equilibrium.

After that, I played the record for him from time to time, sometimes even in group, where everyone seemed to enjoy listening to it. As soon as he heard the beginning of that first song, Frank always expressed his approval with the one word he could say, *gut*, and sometimes he shed a few tears, but he never again exhibited the emotional storm that had overtaken him at his first hearing. Now he often hummed along in his monotone voice.

Like most Alzheimer's patients, Frank had good days and days when he seemed to struggle to stay connected. On good days he was more alert, took note of his environment, and responded to select stimuli. On difficult days he withdrew his attention from his surroundings and did not appear to recognize me or his caregivers as anyone familiar to him. At such times he sat passively through the group session and declined to interact or to engage in the ball-tossing exercises, although that remained his single most satisfying activity for as long as I knew him and worked with him.

Seven months after I first met him and brought him out of his isolation, Frank died in his sleep of a heart attack. His was a merciful death, but I missed him all the same. And I was glad that he had not spent the last months of his life alone in his room.

Chapter 18

One morning upon arriving at the Green Hills Nursing Home, I noticed that the entire staff appeared to be nervous and tense. Everyone went about their tasks with unusual speed and conscientiousness, and without the usual banter staff generally engaged in. In fact, a peculiar silence seemed to have descended on the facility.

Except for those who were confined to bed, all the residents were already up and out of their rooms. They were all immaculately dressed and groomed, with every hair in place. Not a single food-splattered bib was to be seen on any of them. Normally there were always a few residents whose aides had forgotten to remove these after breakfast, or hadn't yet found the time to do so. No one's stockings were falling down, and no one was wearing a sweater inside out or a blouse that hadn't been buttoned correctly.

All the residents' beds had already been made and their rooms put in order. The group of nurses that usually met for a coffee break on the patio at this time was either at the nurses' station, writing frantically in the medical charts, or supervising the aides and making sure that everyone was attending to their assigned duties. It appeared that no one was taking a coffee break today. All of this was highly unusual. It was not yet nine o'clock.

When I entered the area where I normally met with my group,

I found that my residents had already been seated. As I greeted them, a quick scan around the circle informed me that every one of the participants was present and accounted for.

This too, was unusual. In fact, it had never happened before. Usually I had to round up most of them myself. Sometimes I even had to plead with the aides to get my people ready so that I could start my group on time. The CNAs were also supposed to assist in bringing the residents to the designated area, but few of them did so unless they had been late in getting them dressed.

I had just returned from a two-week vacation that day, and I was mystified at all the unusual behaviors I had been observing—but not for long. One of the nurses rushed up to me and whispered in my ear, "HRS is on the premises."

No wonder everyone on staff was on edge. I had been present at another facility when HRS (the state Health and Rehabilitation Services) auditors came to conduct their annual inspection. I knew the auditors would be on the premises for the next several days. They would observe the employees of every department in the performance of their respective duties. They would examine the premises for possible violations of the safety codes. They would read every single entry in a number of randomly chosen medical charts, looking for errors of omission or commission. In short, they examined every aspect of the operation of the facility and the quality of care being rendered. While these inspections are necessary to assure the safety and welfare of nursing home residents, they are also disruptive of the daily routines of the facilities while they are in progress, and they take their toll on the nerves of the staff.

In general, most auditors (there may be as few as three or as many as five) are polite and respectful of the nursing home staff. And they make an effort not to interfere with the caregiving routines. Nevertheless, it is indisputable that these inspections do interfere, to some degree, not only while they are in progress, but often long before they occur as well.

HRS inspects each nursing home once a year, but these inspections do not necessarily take place in the same month every year. In some instances, as many as fifteen or sixteen months can pass between inspections. Facilities are not officially notified of the inspection date, the intention being that the inspectors arrive unannounced so as to prevent the facility from making special preparations designed to make them look better than they really are. But in fact, facilities are rarely caught by surprise.

First of all, before the year has passed and another inspection is due, virtually every facility prepares for the next one well in advance by making all necessary repairs, reviewing all of their caregiving procedures, and sprucing up the place wherever it is needed to meet state regulations. Extra nurses and CNA's often are hired to bolster the regular staff. (In many nursing homes, the number of caregivers is the bare minimum allowed by law, or even fewer).

The fire department is called in to check out the facility and to conduct a fire drill with the staff. (A fire drill is usually a part of the site inspection as well). All medical charts are reviewed (some facilities hire private auditors to do these reviews), and everyone on staff who is responsible for documentation is directed to keep their notes up-to-date. This last requirement involves every department (the DON, the social workers, nurses, physical and occupational therapists, the dietitian, recreation personnel, the attending physicians, etc.).

Now, it is a fact that in every facility where I worked, just about everyone was always behind in their paperwork. It is also a fact that there is simply not enough time in the workday for any of the nursing home staff to keep up with their documentation requirements on a daily basis. Most of the staff worked many uncompensated overtime hours each week to catch up. Those who were unwilling or unable to do this had less time to devote to the residents, and this was unfair to them.

Of course, keeping the medical charts completely up-to-date daily is a state requirement. Any omissions or late entries will result in a citation by the inspectors, if discovered, and this is detrimental to the facility's reputation. No one ever wanted to be the cause of such an outcome. Therefore in the weeks prior to a state inspection, everyone is under stress. One cannot say to oneself, "I will come in on the weekend to catch up," or, "I will stay late tomorrow evening." No, that is not an option when the state inspectors could walk in the next day.

In reality, it is usually only the first facility visited in a given area that is surprised by the arrival of the inspectors. The auditors tend to inspect all the facility in a given city or town, one after another. Within hours after their arrival at the first facility on their list, all the other facilities in the area know that "the state" is in town. Staff in the different facilities know and are friendly with each other and keep each other informed. Administrators of various facilities also often share information.

Naturally, as soon as it becomes known that HRS is near, the collective tension of the staff is heightened and remains high until HRS arrives. In fact it does not abate until the inspectors have gone and the facility has received a good report with only minor infractions cited or none at all. All of the facilities where I worked, both in Florida and New York, consistently received "superior rating" from their respective state inspectors.

It should be noted, however, that just because state auditors sit in positions of judgment of nursing home care, it should not be assumed that all of them are experts in every facet of residential care. From what I have observed, at least some of them are not as knowledgeable as they should be about Alzheimer's disease and about what is appropriate care for this special population.

That morning at Green Hills, after I had completed the group therapy session and had seen several of my other clients individually, I went to the patio to write progress notes and to eat my lunch there.

I had just finished the last of my notes, and was unwrapping my sandwich, when one of the auditors approached me and asked if she could speak with me for a moment. This lady had been introduced to me earlier by the nursing director and had observed a portion of my group session with the Alzheimer's residents. I invited her to sit down, and she told me that she was very impressed by our work. She commented that she thought the MHNH program was a much-needed and wonderful service. "It definitely fills a great gap in residential care," she said.

Naturally, I was pleased by her observation and comments. I knew that our mental health agency was also subject to regular audits by HRS. We had not had an audit since I started my job with the agency, but we were due for one soon. And it would be the first one since the creation of the MHNH program. Therefore, with our agency facing the prospect of HRS scrutiny, I was somewhat reassured that the first auditor who had observed a segment of the program had expressed approval.

We had a pleasant conversation. The auditor ("Call me Janine") expressed an interest in hearing more about MHNH, in particular about our work with Alzheimer's patients. "It must be a challenge to work with these people," she said.

I assured her that it was. Suddenly, she leaned across the table and said, "I need to talk to you about something that really shocked me a little while ago," and she related the following incident.

She had just been to the West Wing (the Alzheimer's unit), to observe lunch being served to the residents.

"Can you imagine, I saw one of the residents, who should have been fed by a staff person, sitting at a table all by herself and lapping food out of a bowl, just like a dog.

"When I protested to the nursing supervisor that this was uncivilized and unacceptable, she told me that this woman always eats like that. That she prefers it that way. She even had the temerity to say that it's a resident's right to choose how she wants to eat."

The auditor was quite indignant.

"Well, I never heard such a lame excuse. After all, this resident has Alzheimer's disease. She's no longer capable of making an informed decision about anything," she continued, "I told that supervisor it has to stop. Someone has to feed this resident from now on."

Janine then asked me to keep an eye on the situation. The implication seemed to be that I should notify HRS if the staff did not comply with her request. I told the auditor that I would check into it, but did not make any other comment. I felt extremely uncomfortable that this woman was confiding in me something that would, undoubtedly, lead to a citation of "resident neglect" in the auditor's report.

Although I had, so far, heard only one side of the story, my sympathy and loyalty lay with the facility. I knew the staff at this facility to be exceptionally caring and conscientious. There had to be a valid reason why this resident was eating her food out of a bowl, as had been described.

As soon as the auditor left the patio, I wrapped up what was left of my sandwich and headed for the West Wing. I spoke to Lilly, the nursing supervisor. I told her about the auditor's conversation with me.

"This is a no-win situation for us, "Lilly commented, already upset.

I asked her who the resident was whose manner of eating had so offended the auditor, and Lilly informed me that it was Alberta D.

I knew Alberta. She was ninety-one years old. She was severely cognitively impaired, physically fragile, wheelchair bound, blind, and unable to communicate verbally. I had been seeing Alberta regularly for sensory stimulation.

She had initially been assigned to my group sessions with Alzheimer's residents, but the very first time she attended, she had become so agitated that she had to be taken out. The staff told me that Alberta was supersensitive to auditory stimuli and needed a very quiet environment. She responded well to one-to-one interactions, but became agitated in any group situation.

"Alberta has no teeth and refuses to wear her dentures. She gets her food pureed and served in a bowl," explained Lilly. "And she absolutely insists on eating by herself. Believe me, we have tried many times to feed her, but she gets very upset if we interfere with her eating. She can no longer hold a spoon because of her contracted fingers, but she does manage to pick up her bowl in her splinted hands and lap the food out of it."

"Do you want to see how she does it?" Lilly asked, then added, "She is still eating her lunch. It takes her a long time to eat, but she is incredibly patient."

We found Alberta seated by herself at one of the tables in the small dining room reserved for residents who had to be fed. An aide was sitting at the next table feeding another resident with a spoon.

Alberta was clutching her bowl in both fists and bringing it to her mouth. The bowl was nearly empty, and she was struggling to get the last of its contents into her mouth with her tongue. Her face had almost disappeared into the bowl.

She barely took note of us as we said "hello." She was totally focused on getting the last morsel and licking the bowl clean. When she was done, she smacked her lips, set the bowl carefully on the table, and gave a grunt of satisfaction.

"My, Alberta, this bowl is as clean as a whistle," exclaimed Lilly.

"I concede it doesn't look civilized," said Lilly, as we walked back to the nurses' station a few minutes later. "But look, this way she eats 100 percent of her meals. To us, that's more important than how it looks. If we try to spoon-feed her, she fights us so hard that half the food ends up on the floor. What's the harm in letting her eat as she wishes? It's not as if we abandon her. There is always an aide nearby who makes sure she's OK and that she drinks her milk and her water."

The next morning, I went looking for Janine, the auditor, and found her seated in the conference room where she was examining medical charts. I asked for a few minutes of her time at her convenience. She put down her pen and invited me to sit down. In spite of the fact that her invitation was accompanied by a kindly smile, I felt like the proverbial mouse in the lion's den.

I told her that I had observed Alberta eating her lunch just as she had described it, and I acknowledged that it did indeed look uncivilized. But I went on to explain to her, as diplomatically as I could, why I thought that the nursing home staff had made the right decision in allowing Alberta to eat her meals without staff assistance.

"Eating her food by herself is the only activity Alberta can still perform by herself," I explained. "When Alberta fought off the staff's attempts to spoon-feed her, she was defending the last shred of independence she still possesses."

OBRA[1] has mandated nursing homes to support the remaining capabilities of the Alzheimer's residents. In manipulating her bowl of food as she did and using her tongue to get the food into her mouth, Alberta was making an extraordinary effort to overcome her disabilities so that she could eat independently. If anything, such effort ought to be applauded and, at the very least, needs to be supported.

Fortunately, Janine proved to be a reasonable person. She not only thanked me for my prompt attention to the situation she had found so shocking, but she also accepted my explanation that in Alberta's case, the facility staff was acting in the best interest of the resident. Contrary to the expectations of the nursing home, HRS did not cite the caregivers for patient neglect.

To judge the behavior of an impaired person by the same standards that we apply to unimpaired members of society is ludicrous. Observing Alberta, I was in awe of her adaptive ability, her tenacity, and her desire to maintain her independence to the extent that was possible.

---

1. OBRA (Omnibus Budget Reconciliation Act), The Nursing Home Reform Legislation, enacted by U.S. Congress 1987 and implemented 1990.

*Oh, I don't eat here, my dear. I just come here to visit my friends,
then I go home to eat with my husband and my son.*

—Gertrude

Chapter 19

The first HRS inspection at which I was present had taken place at Magnolia Manor. Although I worked primarily on the weekend there, I had been asked to help out during the week the inspection was in progress. At the time I was ignorant of the importance of these inspections, but I will always remember an incident that had been rather amusing to observe.

As part of the inspection, the auditors always interview several residents and ask them a variety of questions regarding the care they are receiving and their level of satisfaction with the facility and the staff. If a resident is unhappy and/or voices any complaints, the auditors are very conscientious, requesting immediate correction, and following up to make certain that the problem has been resolved. In a facility that houses alert and oriented residents along with those who are cognitively impaired, HRS generally confines their interviews to alert and oriented residents who can competently answer their questions.

In a facility that caters exclusively to Alzheimer's residents, such as Magnolia Manor, the process of interviewing residents is much more problematic, due to the fact that all of the residents are cognitively impaired, and the majority of them are severely impaired. The auditors therefore look for residents who are the least impaired and, it is hoped, can appropriately answer simple questions regarding the quality of their care and their comfort at the nursing home.

As has been noted in earlier chapters, many of the residents in the early and even in the midrange of AD continue to retain good language and social skills. They also still take an interest in their appearance and are usually well groomed. Many of the women wear jewelry and, like the queen of England, won't be seen anywhere without their handbags. In short, they look like what we think of as "normal." Most of these residents are eager for companionship and enjoy social interaction with others. They are ready to declare their friendship for anyone who smiles at them and offers a friendly greeting.

Gertrude fit that description to a T. In fact, Gertrude stood out in any crowd as someone of distinction. She came from a wealthy family who continued to supply her with elegant and obviously expensive clothes. Her family had arranged for a beautician to come to the nursing home twice a week to attend to Gertrude's hair and nails, even though the facility had a hairdresser on the premises five days per week, and the CNAs took care of the residents' nails.

Gertrude's diction and vocabulary were a notch above everyone else's, and testified to a superior education. Although she was having some problems finding the appropriate word here and there, for the most part her verbalization was usually still within normal range. The content of her communication, however, ranged from the appropriate to the bizarre, depending on the subject and the complexity of the conversation, and also on her ability to process what was asked or communicated to her by others.

Like most Alzheimer's patients, Gertrude could not retain or remember experiences or information of recent or immediate past, and she had great gaps in her memory relating to the past decade or even further back. However, most of the time, on short acquaintance, she gave the impression of being entirely competent.

To the HRS auditor, Gertrude appeared to be the ideal candidate for an interview, and Gertrude herself was only too eager to sit down and have a conversation with this nice lady who had expressed such interest in her.

The interview got off to a good start as the auditor complimented Gertrude on her beautiful dress and her pretty hair. The auditor proceeded to her questions by asking Gertrude how she was feeling. Did she like it here, did she have any friends? Gertrude answered all of these questions appropriately and graciously.

"Thank you, I am very well.

"Yes, I like it very much. It's a nice place.

"Oh yes, I have lots of friends here."

The auditor's next question was, "Is everyone here doing a good job taking care of you?"

To which Gertrude answered, "No one needs to take care of me. I take care of myself."

"I see," said the auditor, "and how do you like the food here?"

"Oh, I don't eat here, my dear. I just come here to visit my friends, then I go home to eat with my husband and my son," Gertrude explained.

There was a moment of silence, then the auditor conducted a brief mental status evaluation. She asked Gertrude, "What day of the week is it? What is today's date? What year is it? Who is the president of the United States?" etc.

Gertrude answered all of these questions incorrectly. When the auditor corrected her, Gertrude nodded her head and said, "Oh yes, dear, I know that, I just forgot." Then came the question, "Where do you live?" Gertrude responded, "I live in Edgewater."

"No, dear," corrected the auditor, "You live here at Magnolia Manor. Don't you remember?"

Gertrude shook her head, impatiently. "I told you, I live in Edgewater at 23 Sunny Lane."

The auditor continued to try to convince Gertrude that she lived at Magnolia Manor. "Look, dear, your room is just down the hall," she said.

With equal insistence Gertrude continued to reply, "You are wrong, I live in Edgewater."

Finally Gertrude had had enough. She got up from her chair and walked away in disgust. Before she turned the corner, on her way to the dayroom, she paused, looked back over her shoulder at the auditor, and stated with immense dignity, "Lady, you don't know anything." Then she disappeared from view.

In Gertrude's mind, there was no clear distinction between past and present. When anyone mentioned home to her, it meant Edgewater, where she had lived most of her adult life. In her perception, she was only visiting her friends in the nursing home.

This frequently caused a problem, especially in the evening when it was time to eat dinner, and later, when it was time to get ready for bed. It required much effort and creative thinking on the part of the caregivers to get Gertrude to consent to cooperate. Reasons had to be given that were acceptable to Gertrude as to why she was going to eat and sleep at the nursing home.

HRS had requested that the nursing home provide a program of reality orientation for the residents. Such programs are, without question, beneficial for those residents who are in the early stages of Alzheimer's disease and for the victims of other types of dementia who have suffered only mild to moderate cognitive and memory impairments. But it simply does not work and would not be appropriate for the residents at Magnolia Manor, all of whom where severely impaired.

The facility did, in fact, practice a brief orientation to reality each morning by way of an announcement at breakfast time and again at the beginning of the morning's recreation programs, e.g., "Good morning, everyone! Today is Monday, June 26, 2000. The sun is shining and it is going to be a warm and beautiful day." However, even that brief bit of reality was meaningless to the residents, except for the brief moment when the information was conveyed. If one asked any of the residents, even five minutes after the announcement, to recall the day's date, or the day of the week, none of them could do it.

The auditor used poor judgment when she insisted on trying to convince Gertrude of the reality of her situation. She only succeeded in upsetting her and making her angry. Gertrude simply did not have the capacity to understand, even though she was still highly articulate in her use of language. In fact, despite her mental impairments, Gertrude had a vast storehouse of knowledge in her memory bank and very detailed recall of past learning and experience up to the time when her son was in his late teens. She recalled that her Edward was a brilliant student and was about to go off to Harvard.

"He is going to be a doctor some day," Gertrude told us frequently, with great pride.

By the time I met Gertrude and worked with her, her son had been a physician for more than twenty years. He had been married and had presented Gertrude with four grandchildren, one of whom was getting ready to go off to college.

But Gertrude did not recognize her grandchildren as such when they came to visit her, nor did she recognize her son. And she no longer had any awareness that her husband had been dead for nearly sixteen years. Alzheimer's disease had robbed her of many of the most rewarding memories of her life, such as the success of her son, the birth and growth of her grandchildren, and precious time spent with her family.

Gertrude could still recite poetry she had learned in school. She remembered her travels in Europe with her parents when she was in her teens. She could recall her student years at Vanderbilt University where she had majored in art history. She often reminisced about that period in her life when she was a student, and she even remembered some of the names of her classmates.

But she could not recall the current season or the day of the week, nor could she remember that she now lived at Magnolia Manor. Most of the time she had no idea whether it was morning, noon, or evening. To insist on reality orientation with such a resident is not only counterproductive, it is cruel.

Validation of perceived reality is a much more appropriate response to the expressed thoughts of a severely cognitively and memory-impaired patient.

Validation therapy was developed by Naomi Feil, MS, ACSW, between 1963 and 1980, in response to her dissatisfaction with traditional method of working with *"severely confused old—old people"* who were her clients.[1]

Using validation, one responds to a confused and/or disoriented person's perceptions without attempting to reason or argue with her. If the person's expressed intentions, actions, or behaviors are contrary to her best interest or have the potential to threaten her health and safety, or that of another person, then caregivers need to use an approach that does not offend the person but gently dissuades and distracts her. In other words, one uses a diversion that captures the confused person's interest and attention. The objective for the caregiver must always be to avoid distressing the resident. A smooth resolution often requires fast thinking, and yes, at times, confabulation as well.

The following chapter will illustrate two such situations in which both validation and confabulation were utilized to preserve a resident's self-esteem and emotional equilibrium.

---

1. Naomi Feil. Biography, Validation Training Institute, Inc. *Validation: The Feil Method,* published in 1982 and *The Validation Breakthrough,* published in 1993, updated and revised in 2002. http://www.vfvalidation.org/feilcv.html

It's my mother's birthday and I have to bake a cake.
We got a lot of company coming.

—Martha

Chapter 20

Martha was a tiny, slender eighty-six-year-old bundle of high energy and good cheer. She had grown up on a farm in Iowa, was married to a farmer when she was seventeen years old, and together they had raised nine children while managing their own large farm.

Martha recalled that she cooked and served three meals a day for her large family and the farmhands. It was not difficult to picture her cooking up a storm, feeding the livestock, milking cows, putting up preserves, and attending to all the other chores required of a farmer's wife.

"We baked all our own bread, biscuits, and pies. We got up before daylight and went to bed with the chickens. We never had much money, but we had a good life," reminisced Martha.

She had been a resident at the Green Hills Nursing Home for three years. Like many of the female residents, Martha has been a widow for more than a decade. She had outlived all but three of her nine children. The surviving members of her family—children and grandchildren—lived in different areas of the country, and none of them were able to take care of her once her Alzheimer's disease had become debilitating.

One morning, as I let myself into the facility's living area, Martha was standing just inside the doorway. She was dressed in several layers of clothing, including her nightgown, two sweaters, and a vest. A baseball cap was perched on her head at a jaunty angle, and her feet were shod in soft felt slippers, down at the heels. She carried a stack of various folded garments in her hands, a stack so high that her head was barely visible above this load.

She greeted me with a broad smile, and said enthusiastically, "Oh good, I'm glad you opened the door so I can get going," as she tried to get past me, out the door.

I continued to stand in the doorway, effectively blocking her escape, and asked her where she planned to go.

"I'm going home, honey. It's my mother's birthday and I have to bake a cake. We got a lot of company coming."

"That's wonderful, Martha," I replied. "How are you going to get there?"

"Honey," said Martha, "My car is right outside. I'm going to drive."

I knew I had to think fast to come up with a reasonable explanation (reasonable to Martha) as to why she could not leave the premises. I recalled that Mary Lucero, in one of her lectures, described a similar incident. She had found a kind explanation, one that was acceptable to the resident. I decided to use the same ruse with Martha.

"Oh Martha," I said, "I forgot to tell you. Your car had two flat tires, and I had the mechanic pick it up to repair them. I'm sorry."

"Oh no," wailed Martha, "How am I going to get home for my mother's birthday?"

"Don't worry, the mechanic promised to bring the car back as soon as it's fixed," I assured her.

Martha was disappointed but accepted this explanation for now, and voiced no objection when I closed the door behind me. I was only momentarily relieved because I knew that I needed to do much more to distract her from her obsession with getting home for her mother's birthday.

I had come to know Martha well in the three years I had been working at Green Hills. Like many Alzheimer's patients in the middle stages of the disease, she had a desire to be helpful to others in any way she could.

"Martha," I said, "I'm going to get the coffee and snacks ready for our group. I really could use some help to set up the trays. Would you be so kind and give me a hand?"

Martha was delighted with my request. Now it was necessary to get rid of the bundle of clothes she was carrying. As long as she had these within sight, they might remind her of her intention to leave, so I suggested we take her clothes back to her room. "You'll need to have your hands free to help me," I told her.

We walked together to her room, and Martha placed the clothes on her bed after refusing my suggestion that she put them back into her drawers. Then I took her to the kitchenette, and she assisted me, as promised.

While Martha was handing out cookies to the group, I managed to convey to one of the CNAs what Martha had been up to that morning. I asked her to inform the nursing supervisor and to have someone go to Martha's room to put her clothes away in her drawers so that she would not have a visual reminder of her intentions to go home. After the snacks had been consumed, Martha helped me to clean up, then participated, as usual, in group. She was very focused on the activities, all of which she enjoyed, and she helped several of her peers to put together the simple puzzles they were working on.

After group I praised her for her assistance, "I couldn't do this job without your help," I told her.

I found other tasks to keep her occupied throughout the day, such as helping me water the plants and visit some of the residents who were confined to bed. In the afternoon I again involved her in group activities. I kept her at my side for most of the day. Not once did she ask about her car or refer to her mother's birthday or needing to get home, at least not for the rest of that day.

If I had applied reality orientation instead of validation of Martha's perception of reality, it would have gone something like this: "Martha, you're eighty-six years old. Your mother is dead.

You are living in a nursing home, and you haven't been able to drive a car for the last fifteen years. The family farm is 1,500 miles from here, and you are not allowed to leave the premises because you are no longer competent to function on your own."

Of course, no one would be so cruel as to say all that to Martha. But I have witnessed, many times, caregivers telling a resident who wanted to exit the premises of a nursing home, "You are not allowed to go out that door," or words to that effect, which provoked immediate anger and agitation

We must remember that those who are cognitively impaired were, prior to the illness, autonomous, able, responsible adults who held jobs, raised children, managed homes, served their communities, and daily made important decisions.

It is true that in the early stages of AD, most victims are aware that they are no longer functioning well, that something is terribly wrong. But once they have reached the later stages in the disease process, they lose this awareness, and once again think of themselves as capable as they were before the illness robbed them of their mental abilities.

So if we tell them, "No, you can't do this—you are not allowed to do that," we, in effect, rob them of their sense of personhood. We diminish their self-esteem. We convey the message that they are our captives, and we are their jailers. How would any of us feel when confronted with such condemnation? Would we not fight and do everything we could to outsmart our captors?

In applying the method of validation in our interactions with Alzheimer's patients, we convey the messages: "I hear you—I value and respect you. I am mindful of your feelings."

There are some experts in gerontology who do not approve of the utilization of untruth in order to resolve problems that arise from a person's misperception of reality, such as Martha's belief that she was needed at home to prepare for her mother's birthday party. But I believe, as do many others who work with Alzheimer's patients, that there is nothing unethical about resorting to fabrication or subterfuge if it serves to spare a patient's feelings and/or prevents a situation from becoming seriously confrontational. What truth is there that would have convinced Martha to give up her intention of walking out the door?

One cannot expect a person to behave reasonably when that person is no longer able to differentiate reality from misperception and delusional thought processes. A caregiver's primary objective must be to resolve problematic situations in such a way that it does not invalidate the patient or engender negative and painful emotions for him or her.

In one of her lectures, Mary Lucero related the following interaction she had with a resident who needed to be rescued from feelings of humiliation. At the time of the incident, Mary was the administrator of a nursing home in Florida.

One day, as she was walking through the Alzheimer's unit of her facility, she came upon a resident who had wet herself but denied that she needed a change of clothes. Not only did the resident refuse, point-blank, to have her clothes changed, but she denied vehemently, and indignantly, that she had wet herself. Mary, realizing that this resident was never going to concede that she had had an accident, and concerned for the woman's hygiene and comfort, as well as for her dignity, quickly got a cup of warm water and spilled it, as if by accident, on the resident's lap.

She then exclaimed loudly, remorsefully, "Oh my, I am so clumsy. Look what I've done to you! I have spilled water all over your clothes. I am so sorry. Please forgive me and let us help you out of these wet clothes."

Since Mary had taken the blame for the resident's wet clothes, the latter made no further objection to having them changed.[1]

One of OBRA's mandates to nursing homes is to "preserve the dignity of the Alzheimer's patient."[2] Another is to "provide comfort care and reassurance."[3] Mary Lucero met both of these mandates admirably with this resident, as I am certain she did with all the residents with whom she came in contact.

If you were to ask yourself, "How do I expect others to treat me?" The answer would likely be the same for each of us: "With respect and courtesy." That is the bottom line in our interactions with each other as civilized human beings. In our interactions with Alzheimer's patients, the aim is the same, but in order to achieve it effectively, we must take the person's mental impairments and altered perceptions into consideration. Validation of perceived reality is one of the tools caregivers can use to assure that the person's self-esteem and dignity are not violated.

---

1. Mary Lucero, Lecturer: *Creative Intervention with the Alzheimer's Patient,* Videotape Lecture (Winter Park, Florida: Geriatric Resources, Inc., 1992).

2. OBRA, Nursing Home Reform Bill, enacted by the U.S. Congress in 1987, implemented in 1990.

3. ibid.

Without memory I am unknown to myself,
lost in an anxiety of darkness.

—Thomas DeBaggio
Losing My Mind[1]

Chapter 21

Madeline was still a beautiful woman at the age of eighty-three. She had large expressive blue eyes, a remarkably clear complexion, and a spectacular mane of long white hair, which she wore pulled back from her face and fastened into a ponytail that cascaded down her back.

Her body was slender and her movements graceful. Although she spent most of her day seated in a wheelchair, she was still able to walk short distances. On any given morning or late afternoon, one could observe her walking along the hallway of Pine Grove, pushing her wheelchair in front of her for exercise. She was determined to maintain her mobility for as long as she could.

Madeline had been married to a handsome U.S. Air Force pilot shortly before the United States entered WWII. A large framed photograph of the young couple was displayed on her bedside table. It had been taken the day before her husband's departure, with his squadron of fighter planes, to the war zone in the Far East.

In the portrait they both looked as glamorous as movie stars, she, with her long blond hair framing her lovely face, wearing an elegant dress dotted with tiny sprigs of flowers, he, in his dashing Air Force uniform, displaying the insignia of a captain. It was the kind of portrait that spoke of love and the promise of a wonderful shared future. But it was not to be. The young husband perished in the Pacific Ocean, somewhere east of Okinawa when his plane was shot down just weeks before the end of the war.

Madeline went to work as a nurse in the pediatric ward of a hospital in Boston. Although she had hoped to have children some day, she never married again. As she once confided to me, "My husband was so wonderful, I just never met another man who could hold a candle to him."

She devoted herself to her work until she was forced to retire at age sixty-one, due to increasing health problems.

When she was admitted to the nursing home at seventy-nine, she had only one surviving relative, her sister, Caroline, who lived in Illinois and was herself too frail to travel and visit Madeline. But they did keep in touch by telephone and via letters.

When I first met Madeline, she was not eligible to participate in the mental health program. She was neither depressed nor cognitively impaired. In fact, she was one of the most well-adjusted nursing home residents I had ever met.

She attended most of the daily recreation programs and participated in every activity the nursing home offered. She particularly enjoyed the crafts hour and proved to be adept at everything she attempted. She was well liked by her peers and had established warm friendships with several women with whom she played Scrabble. She was much admired for the beautiful afghans she knitted, which she gave away to peers.

From the day I arrived at Pine Grove I had many pleasant encounters with Madeline. Whenever she saw me walking down the hall on my way to see my clients, she rushed up to me, in her wheelchair, to fill me in on the latest happenings at the nursing home. She seemed to know everything that occurred.

"Mary fell and broke her hip last night. They took her to the hospital."

"Charlie is being transferred to a place in Philadelphia that's close to where his daughter lives."

"Nurse Anja had her baby. It's a boy."

"Ida got mad at dinner last night and threw her plate full of food on the floor. It was a mess."

Madeline enjoyed telling me all the news before anyone else had a chance to do it. But she also enjoyed sharing reminiscences about her own life. One of the first things she did when we met was to invite me to come to her room so she could show me the portrait of herself and her husband. She often talked about her happy marriage that ended so tragically. But she never dwelled on the sad periods of her life. She had loved her work with sick children during her years as a pediatric nurse.

Sometimes it was difficult for me to have to cut our conversation short, but Madeline understood when I told her that I needed to get on with my work.

She was almost entirely self-sufficient within the nursing home setting in spite of the severe osteoarthritis that confined her to her wheelchair. She needed staff assistance only with bathing and washing her long hair.

She did have occasional short episodes of confusion and disorientation. At such times she had difficulty finding the location of her room, and she would wheel herself frantically up and down the hallway, becoming more and more agitated until one of the caregivers noticed her distress and directed her. She never asked for assistance. Most likely she didn't want anyone to know that she had these little spells.

Within a year of my acquaintance with her, Madeline's episodes of confusion increased, and she began to exhibit other signs of decline in her ability to function. She began to have problems expressing herself verbally. At the same time the recreation staff noticed that her skills in crafts were diminishing. Things that she had always been able to do effortlessly now required immense concentration. Soon she gave up making afghans, as knitting had become a task that was too complex for her. Even such simple projects as stringing beads were a challenge.

Madeline also became confused when she played Scrabble and kept her friends waiting for extended periods of time while she struggled to form the letters in front of her into words that would fit with what was already on the board. When the other players expressed annoyance and impatience, Madeline would throw down her letters in frustration and leave in the middle of a game. Her friends did not understand her behavior. They accused her of being rude and inconsiderate.

Before long, the rules of Scrabble became incomprehensible to Madeline, and she could no longer play at all. Gradually she withdrew from all the activities she used to enjoy. As her language skills diminished, she also avoided social interaction with others. At about the same time, she gave up her daily exercises, and when staff reminded her to walk, she made it clear that she did not feel like making the effort to get out of her wheelchair.

She had by now been enrolled in the MHNH program and attended the daily cognitive and sensory stimulation group sessions. But her attention span was short, and she became exceedingly restless and frequently left the session before it ended. She now sat in her wheelchair the entire day, but rarely remained stationary and spent much time roaming the hallways. That in itself was not a bad thing. Propelling her wheelchair forward, and keeping it in motion, required her to expend energy and provided her with a certain amount of exercise.

Roaming the hallways is an activity that is engaged in by many Alzheimer's patients. Those who are ambulatory spend hours each day pacing back and forth without stopping, and it is frequently necessary for staff to intervene to prevent such residents from becoming totally exhausted.

This restless pacing by Alzheimer's patients has been labeled "sundowning," as most of the pacing takes place in the late afternoon and early evening, although at the nursing homes one sees pacers at any time of the day and night.

Sundowning is an interesting phenomenon. No one knows for

certain what causes this behavior, but there has been much speculation about it. Some caregivers have characterized sundowning as "purposeless activity," but others, myself included, have come to believe that there is a reason and a purpose for the behavior.

It is a fact that people who do not have AD, or any other affliction, engage in pacing under certain circumstances. Prisoners pace in their cells. Professors pace in the classroom while they are lecturing. Students pace while they are memorizing material for tests. Others pace while waiting for someone who is late for an appointment, or when they are trying to come to terms with bad news or are mentally engaged in problem solving, etc. We all pace at times for a variety of reasons.

The only difference between Alzheimer's patients and the rest of us is that we don't, as a rule, do it daily or for prolonged periods of time. And most of us will stop pacing before we reach a state of exhaustion. On the other hand, an Alzheimer's patient is usually unable to stop on his own and needs to be rescued and diverted to a more restful activity.

Wheeling herself around the hallways in her wheelchair was Madeline's way of pacing, and she too needed rescuing after a reasonable time. She was usually quite amenable to being taken to the dayroom to watch TV for a while, or to engage in sorting and folding small laundry items, such as napkins, socks, and washcloths, an activity she now found satisfying.

Madeline's pacing became a problem only when she experienced one of her episodes of anxiety. During those times, she tended to pick up speed and to indiscriminately ram her wheelchair into walls or into the counter of the nurses' station. Anyone who happened to be in the vicinity was at risk of being rammed as well.

Whenever caregivers noticed her on one of her rampages, they would stop her, pull her to the side of the nurses' station, lock the brake on her chair, and admonish her not to move until she had calmed down and regained control.

This strategy rarely, if ever, worked. More often it upset Madeline even more, and at the first opportunity, when she was no longer being observed, she released the brake and was off again, ramming her chair into walls and people. At such times, whichever MHNH staff was on the premises was called upon for crisis intervention.

It was not at all difficult to get Madeline to calm down. Her out-of-control behavior was a signal that she was experiencing emotional distress. She did need someone to stop her behavior as one would stop a runaway train. But it was not enough to pull her aside, tell her not to move—as the caregivers did—and then walk away from her without helping her to regain her emotional equilibrium.

What Madeline needed at such times was someone to spend time with her to comfort and reassure her. Although she could not verbalize what had triggered her distress, she was always highly responsive to personal attention and emotional support. The disease had by now progressed to the point where Madeline lived, so to speak "in the moment," and all her attention and awareness were focused on the present. As soon as she saw a friendly face, heard a reassuring voice, and felt a gentle touch upon her hand, she forgot, instantly, that she had been upset, and it was easy to redirect her attention and engage her in one of the simple activities she could still pursue and that had a calming effect on her, such as stacking plastic dishes in a wire basket or arranging plastic flowers in a container or sorting and folding small laundry items.

It was one of the constant challenges of our work with Alzheimer's patients to discover what would be most helpful in reducing or eliminating their episodes of distress and to return them to their emotional comfort zone. As the residents' physical, cognitive, and emotional status changed over time, caregivers needed to adapt their approaches and strategies to meet changing needs.

AD is known as a disease that, in most cases of late onset (after age sixty-two), progresses relatively slowly. Patients may survive twenty years or more after onset of the disease. I have worked with many residents whose condition remained quite stable during the years I knew them. But I also worked with residents in whom the disease progressed at a rapid pace.

Unfortunately, Madeline was one of the latter. In fact, hers was the most accelerated pace of deterioration I had ever witnessed. And it was especially painful to watch because when I had first met her, she was functioning so exceptionally well.

When she could no longer perform any of her ADLs, Madeline stubbornly resisted staff at every turn, and it became a daily struggle for her CNAs to get her washed, groomed, and dressed, to persuade her to eat her meals, and to get her ready for bed in the evening.

She now spent less time roaming the halls and more time in her room rummaging around in her drawers and closet, shifting things, taking them out, and then putting them back in a messy jumble. It became impossible for her aides to keep Madeline's clothes and underwear organized and neatly stored.

We provided her with a box of things to sort and fold in the hope that she would keep herself occupied with these items and leave her own clothes alone, but that strategy no longer worked. She simply dumped the items out of the box and mixed them with her own things. She seemed to be always a step ahead of her caregivers.

Soon she refused to stay in the dayroom or in the activity room whenever staff set her up there with her laundry basket, or whatever other activity they were trying to interest her in pursuing. It was useless. Within minutes Madeline would wheel herself back to her room to create renewed disorder. To make it worse for the aides, she often took items of her clothing and dropped them in various places around the unit, either in the hallway or in someone else's room. Several times she was observed throwing her clothes into the wastebasket in the dayroom.

At about this time, she also started to go into the rooms of her peers to abscond with anything that came in sight and attracted her attention. One day I intercepted her as she was wheeling herself down the long hallway with a large potted plant in her lap that she had taken from another resident's room. It must have cost her some effort to lift the heavy pot onto her lap.

Another time she had literally cleaned out the chest of drawers of a resident whose room was adjacent to hers. A nurse discovered her in the act of pushing everything under the bed. She had gotten out of her wheelchair and had seated herself on the floor to do this.

Madeline was incredibly resourceful and inventive in creating all sorts of disorder on her unit, and she kept the caregivers occupied with damage control. There is no doubt that their work was made unreasonably more stressful because there were simply not enough caregivers per shift to attend to the kind of challenging and needy residents they had on this unit.

To make matters worse, Pine Grove was one of those nursing homes where alert and oriented residents lived on the same unit as the dementia residents and there was constant friction because the latter invaded the rooms of the former and often took their belongings or even lay down on their beds.

More and more frequently I, or one of my staff, was paged to do an intervention with Madeline or one of the other residents who were acting out. Madeline was not the only Alzheimer's resident on the unit whose behaviors were inappropriate at times. Often several altercations between residents were going on at the same time, and the staff was hard-pressed to sort out the problems, soothe injured feelings, and restore peace on the unit.

Madeline continued to attend the CSS program five times per week. She was now primarily responsive to one to one attention. Her language skills had dwindled to single words, but she could still comprehend the simple commands and follow the cues we demonstrated for the group during the exercise segment of the session. She could no longer join in the singing, but she loved to clap hands in time to the music. She still enjoyed folding small laundry items, although she no longer sorted these, as she had done earlier.

Then, seemingly in the blink of an eye, the disease progressed to another level. Madeline became withdrawn; her attention span and her ability to remain focused on anything could be counted in seconds. Speech—even single words—were no longer possible for her; her speech had been reduced to incoherent babble.

In group she ceased to participate and spent the hour picking at her clothes. Soon she became completely indifferent to her surroundings and no longer recognized any of her caregivers. We had all become strangers to her.

Her body as well as her mind began to fail as the disease drew the last bit of strength and muscle tone from her. She began to slump forward in her wheelchair, and a lap tray was secure to the front of it to prevent her from falling out. When her torso began to list to the left side and she could no longer hold up her head, she was placed in a recliner chair. It was a shock to see Madeline looking so small and shrunken in that big chair. She had slipped into the next and final stage of AD.

She continued to have episodes of distress when she cried out and slammed her fists against the sides of her chair. Her eyes were tightly shut and her face contorted. The sounds that issued from her mouth were like those an infant in need of comforting. The staff were used to hearing them several times a day and no longer reacted to them since Madeline did not respond to their attempts to soothe her. She was one of several residents on the unit whose voices were raised in repetitious sounds. But some of the alert and oriented residents protested loudly about the disturbance created by Madeline, especially when she was place in the dayroom, where they were trying to watch TV. At the next care-plan review meeting for Madeline it was decided to keep her in bed, where she now appeared to be most comfortable.

Whenever I came to see her and found her in a state of restlessness or agitation, I simply gathered her up in my arms and rocked her, as one would rock an infant, until she stopped trembling and her tortured voice ceased. I held her and rocked her and hummed one of the nursery rhymes she used to sing to the sick children in the pediatric ward. I rocked her till her body relaxed and she became so heavy in my arms that I could not hold her any more. Then I gently laid her back on her pillow and stroked her brow until she fell asleep. It was all I could do for her now. One morning when I arrived at Pine Grove, the staff informed me that Madeline had been hospitalized with pneumonia. She died two days later.

---

1. Thomas De Baggio, *Losing My Mind* (New York: Simon and Schuster, 2000), 182.

The first time I grieved for Madeline was on the day I walked into her room and realized that she had no idea who I was anymore.

—Erin, CNA

Chapter 22

When Madeline died, her loss was deeply felt by the caregivers on her unit. Even some of the housekeeping and kitchen staff voiced sadness. But Sandra and Erin, the CNAs who had been taking care of Madeline for many years and had come to love her, expressed the greatest sorrow.

"For me, it's like she died twice," Erin noted, tearfully. "The first time I grieved for Madeline was on the day I walked into her room and realized that she had no idea who I was anymore. It finally dawned on me then that her mind was really gone. We used to have such fun together. She was so easy to take care of, and so proud of all she could still do by herself."

Erin was surprised that Madeline's actual death hit her so hard. She had not expected it. I, too, mourned Madeline's death. I felt particularly sad that she had died in the hospital, without the presence of anyone who loved her—she, who had given so much love and devotion to sick children during the years when she had worked on the pediatric ward of a Boston hospital.

Madeline was one of more than a dozen clients of the MHNH program who had died by that time. Most of these residents had died at the nursing home, and I had been able to spend time with several of them during their last hours. Some of these passings had been more painful for me than others. But no matter how painful the losses of residents we had come to know and cherish, none of us who work in a caregiving capacity at the nursing homes have the luxury of dwelling in mourning, but for a brief time, those who are gone. The very nature of our work demands that we focus our attention on the living, who need us so much.

So when Madeline died, those of us who had been close to her—her CNAs, Sandra and Erin, several of the nurses, and I—got together in the privacy of the medical records storage room at break time to share our grief. With words and tears and a quick hug we comforted each other. Then we composed ourselves and returned to the unit to go about our respective duties.

One of my duties that afternoon was to gather together the group of ladies who had been friends of Madeline's. Jackie, Jean, Melanie, and Madeline (their peers had dubbed them J.J. and M'n M.) used to play Scrabble together every afternoon from four o'clock till dinnertime in the small plant-filled lounge adjacent to the dining room. Madeline had withdrawn from the group after she had become so confused that she could no longer participate in the game.

Now that the friends had learned of her death, they expressed feelings of guilt and regret that they had cut off all contact with Madeline after her condition deteriorated. I reminded them that it was Madeline who had withdrawn from them, and that she would have continued to see her friends if she had felt comfortable doing so.

"Well, I actually did try to talk to her several times after she stopped playing Scrabble with us," explained Jean. "My room is just down the hall from hers. But she didn't seem to know who I was and she just turned away. After that, I never talked to her again."

"Gosh," exclaimed Melanie, "it's so sad what happened to her. We used to have so much fun when Madeline was still part of our gang."

"She was so smart," added Jackie. "She was like a walking dictionary. She had the best vocabulary of any of us. She won most of the games, you know."

"You should have seen some of the words she made," Jackie laughed, remembering, and said in a near whisper, "you know, some of the words she put down on the board were downright naughty." All three of the ladies giggled.

The mood of the group lightened considerably as the friends, one by one, took turns recalling some particularly memorable and amusing experiences they had shared with Madeline. By the time the meeting broke up, all three of the ladies felt better, and so did I.

Many people think of nursing homes as places where the old and sick come to die. And it is true that for the majority of residents, a nursing home is their last abode on this earth. But in reality nursing homes are places that are full of life, where one can observe a broad spectrum of the human condition in old age. Though the residents may be fragile and afflicted with a variety of chronic and debilitating diseases, many of them nevertheless remain actively engaged in life to the extent they are able.

There is usually a core group of residents who are no longer able to live on their own but who thrive within the safety of the nursing home, which takes care of all their physical needs. Many of these residents have maintained—in some cases regained—a capacity to enjoy the companionship of their peers and to participate fully in the social and recreational activities of the facility. Yet sometimes without warning, one or another of these residents is suddenly struck down by a stroke, a heart attack, or some other fatal condition and dies. In the midst of life, death is ever present and often unpredictable.

On the other hand, there are residents who seem to be in constant peril of dying, and yet survive numerous episodes of near-fatal medical crises, hanging on to life, however precariously, year after year.

There are also residents who are on life support systems when they arrive at the nursing home (usually straight from the hospital), and it is understood by the staff as well as by the patient's family that nothing more can be done to prolong life and that death is imminent.

Sometimes, in such cases hospice is called in to keep the patient comfortable and to provide emotional support to the dying person in his or her last days, as well as to the family. However, in the majority of cases it is the nursing home caregivers who tend to the dying resident.

Whether the death of a resident is sudden and unexpected or whether weeks, or months, or years pass before the end comes, the actual death of any resident impacts everyone on the unit, particularly those of his/her peers who had developed a close relationship with the deceased and the staff who have been most closely involved in the resident's care.

During their professional training, caregivers are cautioned not to become emotionally attached to those they care for. It is believed that such closeness would impair their ability and judgment in meeting the care needs of their patients responsibly and appropriately, and furthermore, maintaining professional aloofness will protect them from the pain of loss when patients die. It is further believed that the cumulative effect of such losses would, most likely, adversely affect the caregiver's ability to cope, and may result in early job burnout, particularly for those who work in hospitals and nursing homes. The paradox is that caregivers are expected to provide compassionate, even tender, loving care for their patients while at the same time remaining emotionally aloof.

The truth is that people who are ill, especially those who are confined to nursing homes, whose contact with family and friends are limited, and those who no longer have any surviving family or friends, often become deeply attached to their primary caregivers out of a need for warmth and human connectedness. And it is quite common, indeed natural, that caregivers respond in kind to the affection showered on them by their patients.

A friend of mine who had once been hospitalized for severe depression told me that what helped her most to get well was not the psychotherapy or the medication she received, but the warmth and affection extended to her by the nurses, the nurses' aides, and the recreation staff throughout her hospital stay.

Some caregivers are, by nature, warm and cheerful personalities; others are more reserved and emotionally detached from their patients. However, if truth be told, it is the former type of caregiver who provides the higher quality of care because such caregivers take into account not only the patients' physical-care needs, but their emotional and psycho-social needs as well, and they respond to those needs.

If I were a resident at a nursing home, there is no question that I would prefer to have caregivers around me who have the capacity to relate and respond to my feelings. The very best kind of caregivers are those who can be cool and detached in a crisis but warm and affectionate at any other time. And it also helps if they have a sense of humor.

For those of us who provide mental health services, however, it is considered a breach of ethics to get friendly with a client. There is an ironclad rule in mental health that one cannot be effective in this work unless one can remain objective and keep a formal distance from the client at all times and in all circumstances.

Frankly, I have never met another human being who is entirely objective. We are all influenced in subtle and not-so-subtle ways by the people we meet and interact with, by our innate personalities, life experiences, and environment. And we are, therefore, all subjective in more ways than we are even consciously aware of. Every person, whether psychiatrist, nurse, or fishmonger, brings his or her own personal baggage to every encounter and interaction with others, professional or personal. To deny the reality of this is to live in the land of make-believe.

For every person with Alzheimer's, there are countless others in close proximity who feel and live with the impact of the disease.

—Lisa Snyder, LCSW
Speaking Our Minds[1]

Chapter 23

When we are young, older and wiser folks advise us to save and plan for our retirement and old age so that we will have the resources to see us through the final stages of life in comfort, free of want. But whether or not we heed such advise, most of us envision ourselves in "our golden years" engaged in enjoyable leisure activities—traveling the world, taking up painting, growing orchids—perhaps even starting a new career.

The possibilities seem endless as we contemplate doing all the things for which we never have time during the years when most of our time, and energy are consumed by career and family obligations. In our senior years we will be free of these constraints, and we will live the good life. It will be our reward for all the years we invested in doing what was expected of us. We have earned it.

While we are still young, few of us can conceive of ourselves as so frail and helpless that we have to depend on others to meet our needs. Few of us can imagine ourselves as victims of some dreadful chronic disease that will rob us of a wonderful retirement. It is not that we don't know about the diseases that afflict so many of the elderly; it's just that we need to believe that we ourselves will be spared. To think of the alternative would be just too frightening.

However, as we get older, and especially after we have attained senior-citizen status, most of us give up these delusions of invulnerability, and we begin to concede the possibility that we too may fall victim to an incapacitating illness.

Statistically, Alzheimer's disease is, at present, one of the most prevalent diseases that afflict the elderly. As stated earlier, by age sixty-five, one in ten people has AD, and by age eighty-five nearly 50 percent of that population will be affected.

Anyone with a close relative who has AD—a parent, grandparent, or sibling—knows that a genetic link may put him or her at higher risk for getting the disease. To date, five genetic markers have been identified, one on each of chromosomes 1, 12, 14, 19, and 21. There are now diagnostic tests available that reveal if a person has one or more of these genetic markers for the disease. But it is by no means certain that a person who has one or more of these markers in their genetic code will actually get AD. But there is no doubt that it puts him/her at higher risk.

In addition, medical scientists now tell us that there are many other risk factors that can contribute to the development of the disease, such as having one of the chronic inflammatory diseases, having high cholesterol, high blood pressure and/or neglecting to remain mentally and physically active. So whether or not one gets tested, there is no definitive answer to the question, "Will I get Alzheimer's disease?" The best we can hope for is that medical science will manage to eradicate the disease before it catches up with us.

Scientists in research centers across the United States and in other parts of the world are hard at work to find a cure and/or means to prevent AD. But while they are making progress toward these goals, as of this writing, they have not as yet been successful.

Several medications have been developed, tested, and approved by the FDA that supposedly slow down the disease process in some patients, provided they begin taking the medications in the early stages of the disease. However, these medications are effective only in approximately 50 percent of the patients taking them, and they work only on a temporary basis. It should also be noted that these medications can have serious side effects.

The financial cost of caring for Alzheimer's patients is enormous. The emotional pain the disease imposes on its victims and on their families is immeasurable.

Like everyone else, I have no way of predicting whether or not I will ever become a victim of AD. At age sixty-seven, I am well into the age where the disease is rampant. I don't know of anyone in my family who has or had AD. My paternal grandparents both lived to a ripe old age, well beyond the life expectancy for human beings who had been born in the latter part of the nineteenth century.

My grandmother died of cancer at the age of seventy-three. I do not know what kind of cancer it was, except that it was located in the lower region of the body. Nobody talked about cancer in those days (it was 1942). The subject was as taboo as TB, mental illness, and, of course, anything to do with sex. I wish I had asked my mother, before she died, what kind of cancer it was, but I was still young and healthy, and illness of any kind was not on my mind.

I remember visiting my grandmother at the hospital during the last few days of her life. She looked frail and wasted. I could tell she was very weak, but she was mentally alert and lucid to the end.

My grandfather survived my grandmother by three years. At age eighty-three he fell and fractured his right femur while taking his customary daily walk through the neighborhood. He exhibited some confusion and disorientation thereafter, but this was probably induced by the morphine that had been prescribed for pain. He died of a stroke two months after the accident. He too had been mentally fit and alert before his final illness.

I have no way of knowing if my father would have contracted AD had he survived to old age. He was lost to us at age forty-four, missing in action on the Russian front, during the last year of WWII.

My mother's family history is very different from my father's. On the last day of his life, my maternal grandfather took the train to the city of Pforzheim, where he worked as a goldsmith. At the end of his workday he ran to catch his train home. He managed to climb aboard the last car as the train was pulling out of the station, but he died of a massive heart attack before the train reached his hometown. He was fifty years old.

On the day my maternal grandmother died a year later, she had also taken the train into the city. She had gone to buy some things she could not get in the small village where the family lived. She too ran to catch the train in order to get home in time to cook dinner, and she actually made it all the way home. But when she got there, she told her children that she was not feeling well and went to bed. A few hours later she too was dead of a heart attack. She was fifty-one. At age sixteen my mother was an orphan.

From all that my mother has told me about her parents, I can assume that they were fully functional until the day they died. For me, the moral of their early deaths was "never run to catch a train." And I never did.

Neither did my mother. But she could not escape the family disease, nor did her sisters. Two of her sisters died of heart attacks and one of a stroke, all of them before they reached the age of fifty-five. My mother, the youngest of the siblings, made it to age sixty-seven before she, too, died of a heart attack.

Toward the end of her life, my mother exhibited symptoms of acute paranoia. She believed that the FBI and the Mafia were after her. She used to tell us that every time she went to her bank they watched and followed her. Yet she was able to take care of herself, and even traveled to Europe by herself shortly before she died.

I wonder whether the paranoia could have been a symptom of the onset of Alzheimer's disease. Or was it caused by one of the other diseases of the brain? I'll never know. But I do speculate about it, especially on days when I have misplaced my glasses or my keys, or when I have done something stupid, like forgetting about the rice that was cooking on the stove until I smelled the burned residue in the scorched pot.

Then there are those times when I can't recall the name of an actor in a movie I had recently seen. We used to call such lapses "having a senior moment." Now we are more apt to say "we are having an Alzheimer's moment."

I worry about my mental lapses, because these incidents, however few they are, could be signs of the onset of AD.

Experts in AD tell us that maintaining a healthy lifestyle will reduce the risk factors for the disease. The Alzheimer's Association has recently launched a public awareness campaign and is conducting nationwide workshops called *Maintain Your Brain. How to live a brain-healthy lifestyle.* Their recommendations include adopting a brain-healthy diet, staying physically and mentally active and remaining socially involved.[2]

I am definitely heeding that advice. And whenever I think of it—usually after one of my memory lapses—I engage in a series of mental exercises to test my memory. And when I have to make any kind of calculation, I do it in my head rather than reaching for the calculator.

Yes, I worry about the state of my brain. But I am also good at rationalizing my mental aberrations when they occur. Come to think of it; the ability to rationalize well, to explain mental lapses, is one of the hallmarks of the onset of AD. That aside, I have always been like the proverbial absentminded professor. When I am occupied with a creative project, I tend to be forgetful about all else.

Naturally, I hope that I will live in reasonably good health for many more years, and will continue to be able to take care of myself and maintain my independence. However, I do have to address the possibility that I may, at some future date, become incapacitated by illness, possibly even AD. I feel I owe it to my children to have some concrete plan for such an eventuality so that not all the responsibility falls on them to make decisions regarding my care should I become mentally incompetent.

For as long as I can remember, the prospect of being confined to a nursing home at the end of my life has been abhorrent to me. My first actual visit to such an institution only intensified these feelings.

I will never forget the nursing home to which my mother had been transferred in 1970 from the hospital where she had been treated for her first heart attack. This facility was housed in an old five-story building in a small town in New Jersey. The first time I visited my mother there, when I got off the rickety elevator on the fourth floor, I found myself in a dimly lit room with gray wall and an assortment of shabby furnishings. This was the dayroom.

A group of residents in wheelchairs were lined up against a wall, and several others were seated on a sagging old couch. There was nothing in that room to stimulate the senses or uplift the spirit, and the residents sat silently staring into space. A nurse led me down a long, equally dingy narrow hallway that was lined on either side with small cramped rooms, each containing two beds. The whole scene suggested a rabbit warren.

I found my mother lying in bed looking sad and forlorn. Although it was now past two o'clock in the afternoon, her lunch tray was still sitting on the tray table at her bedside, the food congealed on the plate. The faded curtain was half drawn across a filthy window. It was a dismal place to be. My brothers and I decided to take our mother out of that facility immediately, as it was evident that her condition could only deteriorate in such a depressing environment.

It would be unfair, and probably inaccurate, to characterize all nursing homes of early vintage as being environmentally as bleak as that one was. There is no question that this particular facility was substandard in every respect, including the kind of care the residents received. However, I visited several other nursing homes in New York and Connecticut during that time, and none of these appeared to be much better. They too were shabby, colorless, and cramped, and their residents appeared to be depressed and devoid of animation. A sense of doom and hopelessness pervaded these places, and I remember thinking, "Oh God, please spare me from having to spend my last days on earth in such surroundings."

There were probably some nursing homes that were attractive and comfortably furnished, where the patient care was good, but all too many facilities in those days lacked any redeeming qualities that would have permitted their residents to live out their remaining years being well cared for in a pleasant environment.

Initially, nursing homes in the United States were established to provide custodial care for patients who had suffered serious health crises such as strokes, heart attacks, and other disabling conditions and who needed continued care after release from the hospital. There were also private homes that accepted and cared for frail elderly people who could no longer manage to live independently.

Care in these establishment was basic, and little, if any, emphasis was placed on providing either a cheerful environment or opportunities to engage in activities that offered mental stimulation and relieved boredom.

Prior to the implementation of Medicare and Medicaid in 1965, there were neither federal nor state regulations to set standards and assure that nursing home residents in the United States received quality care and humane treatment. Nor was there any agency in place to monitor and hold individual institutions accountable for the quality of care and services they provided. In fact, it was generally conceded, by persons who had experience with them, that many facilities fell far short of providing even minimally acceptable care.

By 1991, the year I began my work as coordinator of the Mental Health Nursing Home Program, dramatic changes had taken place in nursing home care. The physical environment in most facilities was much improved; gone were the gray walls, bland rooms, and dingy furnishings. Most of the facilities in which I came to work or visit over the next eight years presented attractive, comfortably appointed living quarters. Although the residents' personal rooms continue to be marginal in size, most of the shared living spaces, such as dayrooms, dining rooms, and recreation areas, are spacious and nicely decorated.

Many of the homes also feature beautifully landscaped grounds, some with patios and well-tended footpath, where residents can take a stroll or sit and socialize with their visitors and peers, while enjoying the fresh air.

These days all nursing homes that participate in the Medicare and Medicaid programs are required to provide a full range of rehabilitation services with qualified physical, occupational, and speech therapists, etc., for those residents who can benefit from such services.

Another important development has been the establishment of recreation departments. These offer the residents the opportunity to engage daily in a variety of group and individual activities they enjoy. Such programs also promote mental and physical stimulation, and they encourage and facilitate social interaction among peers.

These improvements came about primarily as a result of OBRA (Omnibus Budget Reconciliation Act), the Nursing Home Reform Legislation enacted by Congress in 1987 and implemented in 1990. The mandates of this bill were to change the focus of nursing home care from the custodial model (as practiced in hospitals and providing basic physical care) to a holistic model of caregiving that is designed to meet the mental, emotional, psychosocial, environmental, and rehabilitative needs of long-term care residents.

In short, these new federal regulations revolutionized the whole concept of caring for the elderly who are confined to nursing homes. The primary goal of this legislation was to improve the quality of care and the quality of life[3] for every resident. The mandate was for each resident to achieve the highest possible level of functioning through restorative care.

Prior to OBRA, nursing home residents were viewed by the general public (as well as by many health-care professionals) as helpless individuals who had reached that stage in life where conditions of frailty and ill health were to be expected and were considered to be a normal feature of the aging process. And it was generally assumed that nothing could be done to improve their conditions or the quality of their lives.

OBRA changed all that. Residents are now encouraged to take part in the development of their care plans and to participate actively in their rehabilitation, to the extent that they are able. They are encouraged to participate in their ADLs (activities of daily living, such as dressing, grooming), and caregivers are charged with assisting them, only as necessary, rather than doing all such tasks automatically for them.

A "Residents' Bill of Rights" is posted in every nursing home, where it is visible to residents, staff, and visitors at all times. According to this bill, the residents are now given choices as to their care—their preferences of daily routine, recreational activities, etc.—and they are to be encouraged to exercise their right to make these choices.

In spite of the many positive changes in the nursing home environment and improvements in the quality of care, there are still many facilities that do not measure up. Even some of the facilities that have consistently received "Superior" rating from state auditors are not necessarily the best choices for a loved one who has Alzheimer's disease. In many facilities caregivers still lack the skills needed to meet the special care needs of their Alzheimer's residents. One must keep in mind that the state's inspections require that the facilities meet only the minimum standards of federal and state regulations. Therefore a "superior" rating is, in some cases, a relative term.

The general public is well aware of the shortcomings of many nursing homes, and although every year more and more Alzheimer's patients are placed in nursing homes, the majority of these patients continue to be cared for at home, usually by members of their families. In most cases the primary caregiver is a spouse, a daughter, or a sibling of the patient.

Having a family member who suffers from AD is a devastating and deeply painful experience for everyone. Taking care of the patient at home is demanding and exhausting in the extreme for the primary caregiver. It is a task that consumes every minute of every day, and often the nights as well. And in most cases, the job goes on for years and years, and it gets harder and harder as the patient becomes increasingly more incapacitated. Such demands can wear out the strongest person physically, emotionally, and spiritually, and it can have a devastating effect on family life.

The final chapter of this book explores the options of care for Alzheimer's patients and provides information concerning practical strategies families can employ to assist and support an afflicted loved one in the early stages of AD, as well as later, when the disease has progressed to such a degree that the patient requires total care.

---

1. Lisa Snyder, LCSW, *Speaking Our Minds, Personal Reflections from Individuals with Alzheimer's* (New York: Freeman and Co., 2000), 5.
2. The Alzheimer's Association quarterly national newsletter, Winter 2005.
3. Federal Regulations, Title 42, Sec. 483.25: Quality of Care. Title 42, Sec. 483.15: Quality of Life. Requirements for Long Term Care Facilities.

Give me hugs, hold my hand and demonstrate your love.

—Ursula

Chapter 24

Until now I have never seriously discussed with my children what should be done if I were to become physically and/or mentally disabled and in need of full-time care. I do recall that over the years I have made pronouncement to the effect that it would be unacceptable to me ever to be placed in a nursing home.

I also recall telling my children, more than once, that were I to become senile, they should encase me in a block of cement and drop me into the Hudson River. Although it was said in jest, it did imply that I did not wish to live once my mental faculties were gone.

In effect, I gave my children just two options in the event of my becoming incapacitated: either to commit matricide or to assume the burden of my care, however difficult that might be, and however long it might disrupt their own lives.

While I have great admiration for family caregivers who have taken it upon themselves to care for a loved one with AD at home, I am well aware of the enormous price they are paying in time and energy. I know with absolute certainty that I do not wish my children to assume such a burden for me. It would break my heart to have their lives—their every waking hour—consumed by the demands of caring for an Alzheimer's patient for what is, in most cases, a prolonged period of time.

However, that does not mean that I expect my children to drop me off at the nearest nursing home the first time they observe me placing my shoes in the refrigerator or showing up at their children's school on Grandparents' Day wearing a sweater inside out over my pajamas.

As stated in an earlier chapter, Alzheimer's is a disease that tends to progress slowly, and the degree of impairments varies from person to person. In the early stages many patients continue to function reasonably well for a time, except for lapses in short-term memory and occasional episodes of confusion, and family members may attribute these to be symptoms of normal aging.

However, when these episodes increase to the extent that the person is having problems managing routine tasks of daily living, it is time for a complete medical checkup and assessment of the person's neurological functioning.

Too many families delay such a checkup for various reasons, not the least of which is to postpone hearing possible bad news, such as a diagnosis of AD. There are many other medical conditions that can cause memory impairments, and other mental aberrations that are also typical of AD. And some of these conditions can be treated, and symptoms of dementia may disappear.

If, however, a diagnosis of dementia of the Alzheimer's type has been established, it is usually as devastating to the family as it is to the patient. It is important for family members to learn all that is known about AD to help them understand what the patient will be experiencing as the disease progresses and what resources are available to assist them and the patient in dealing with the disease. What the patient will need most—and needs immediately—is emotional support from those near and dear, and reassurance that he/she will not be abandoned.

In the early stages of the disease many patients are able to continue to manage routine household chores. Some even continue to live independently in their own homes, at least for a time, and continue to pursue a variety of accustomed activities and interests.

It is just that most tasks will become more challenging and require more concentration and effort.

In time the patient will need to make increasing practical adjustments and accommodations to the cognitive impairments and memory deficiencies as they arise. Many painful decisions will have to be made when activities that represent independence and autonomy have to be relinquished once they become too stressful or difficult for the person to manage any longer. For instance, when the patient experiences episodes of confusion and disorientation, the time has come to give up driving.

When bills pile up and the person has trouble managing finances, it is necessary to let someone else take over the checkbook. Driving a car and managing personal finances are just two of the many skills that an AD patient will eventually lose. And all of these losses will cause emotional distress, embarrassment, and diminished self-esteem.

The patient's family can be of immense assistance in helping him/her deal with and accept the limitations by demonstrating continued support, affection, and respect, while offering practical help where it is needed. But it is also important to allow the patient (and even to encourage him/her) to practice their remaining skills to the full extent.

Most Alzheimer's patients enjoy social interaction with family and friends, although they may withdraw from contact with others as their impairments become more acute. That is one of the means by which they try to hide their episodes of confusion and forgetfulness. Yet many patients are creative in the utilization of adaptive measures to compensate for their memory deficits. They may make lists of "things to do," place labels on closet doors and drawers, and write notes to themselves to assist their failing memories.

Family and friends can do much to help the patient retain self-esteem, first by being nonjudgmental, accepting that the person has special needs, second, by encouraging the patient to remain engaged in daily activities as she/he is able, and to anticipate where and when the person needs a helping hand.

Be patient, be kind. Watch for depression, which is particularly common as the person struggles to deal with failing memory and cognitive loss. Remain calm and supportive when the person becomes upset, agitated, and angry at the problems she/he experiences. Do not add to the person's distress by arguing or by thoughtless comments.

It is important to bear in mind that you are not alone in coping with this disease. There is help out there, and it is recommended that you avail yourself of it. First and foremost, there is the Alzheimer's Association, which has chapters in most communities throughout the country and disseminates a wealth of information on all aspects of Alzheimer's disease. This organization provides assistance and guidance to patients as well as to their families, from the earliest symptoms through the most difficult times ahead. It offers support groups for both patients and family members. The participants are very supportive of one another and have much insight and practical advise to share.

Most communities have established one or more adult day care centers for Alzheimer's patients. These centers offer programs designed to enhance and maintain, for as long as possible, the patient's abilities through a variety of activities, such as cognitive and sensory stimulation exercises, games, crafts, reminiscing, sing-alongs. Most importantly, the participants at these centers enjoy daily social interaction with others who share their problems.

Most of the day care centers offer five-day-per-week programs, and most provide transportation to and from the patients' homes. These programs usually run from nine or ten in the morning until four or five in the afternoon. Nutritious lunches and snacks are provided. The personnel is generally well trained and skilled in meeting the needs of Alzheimer's patients. A registered nurse is on staff at all times to dispense the participants' prescribed medication and to deal with any medical emergencies that may arise.

For those patients who prefer to continue to live independent of their families, yet can no longer manage the more complex tasks of independent living and personal care (shopping, preparing meals, remembering to take their medications, etc.), there are assisted living facilities designed for the mild to moderately cognitively impaired. At these facilities residents live in their own small apartments, furnished, in some cases, to the residents' personal taste and specifications. These facilities offer a variety of support services, such as housekeeping, laundry service, meals, recreation and exercise programs, access to the outdoors in a safe environment, and transportation to stores and medical appointments. There is a registered nurse on staff at all times and a staff trained to supervise and assure the comfort, well-being, and safety of the residents.

These facilities are fairly new, and as yet there are relatively few of these state-of-the-art establishments. They are also quite expensive, but for those who can afford them, they do offer superior alternative accommodations for relatively independent living.

Most families who have a newly diagnosed loved one suffering from Alzheimer's have more questions than answers about the disease. Many will discover that their physicians are not of much assistance in providing advise and support regarding what to expect or how best to cope with the situation. In addition to the Alzheimer's Association, there are several excellent books that can be indispensable at this time. At the end of this chapter, the reader will find a list of such books. Some of these have been written by experts in AD; some were authored by family members of Alzheimer's patients who share their personal experiences of caregiving for a loved one. Last but not least, several of the most moving and insightful books have been written by patients of AD who describe what they are experiencing as they struggle to cope with the impact Alzheimer's has on their lives during the early stages of the disease, while they are still fully aware that something terrible is happening to them. All of these books and many more that are not listed should be of immense help to anyone whose life has been touched by Alzheimer's, be they patients, family members, or professional caregivers.

Inevitably, the time comes for most AD patients when they will no longer be able to survive on their own, when supervision and assistance are no longer adequate and they are in need of total care. Families should decide before the patient reaches this state whether they are able and willing to take on the burden of caring for the patient at home or whether it would be best for all concerned to place the person in a long-term care facility.

The decision to place a beloved family member in a long-term care facility is, for most families, a very painful and emotionally charged issue. Many families harbor feelings of guilt about relinquishing the caregiving to professionals, even when it is obvious that they themselves are unable to continue to care for the patient at home.

It is well documented that in most cases, families wait until they are faced with a crisis or have reached the end of their ability to cope with a seriously ill relative before they begin to consider other caregiving options. This is most unfortunate, because at that point the family is often forced to make a quick decision, under acute stress, without the benefit of comparing different facilities and what they have to offer.

The best time to begin the process of learning about the quality and range of services and amenities offered by different institutions is before the need for placement arises. In order to make an informed decision as to the best and most suitable facility for the patient, it is necessary to visit as many facilities as possible and to ask questions about every aspect of care and services. Of course, it is essential to know what to look for and what questions to ask.

In seeking nursing home placement for an Alzheimer's patient, it is important to choose a facility that is equipped to meet the special environmental and care needs of this population The very best kind of facility in my experience, is one that caters exclusively to Alzheimer's residents, such as Magnolia Manor. As a rule, these facilities have been specifically designed to provide a serene, safe environment in which residents can freely move from area to area, within their unit, without feeling trapped or lost. There is usually easy access to enclosed outdoor areas to give the residents a sense of freedom. The staff is well trained to provide the best of care, and activities are geared to stimulate and keep the residents occupied with purposeful activities that are designed to maintain and enhance the person's remaining abilities for as long as possible (one of the OBRA mandates). Emphasis is placed on assisting the residents in maintaining self-esteem and minimizing feelings of frustration and emotional distress.

Unfortunately, there are as yet relatively few such facilities in most communities, and it may be necessary to settle for a less ideal situation. If so, the next best option is a facility that offers separate units for Alzheimer's patients. Some of these facilities are also a good choice if they have made an effort to meet the special environmental and care needs of the Alzheimer's residents. But one needs to check these facilities carefully. Some of them may offer separate units, but otherwise they do not differ in the services and care they provide, and it should not be assumed that the staff in the Alzheimer's unit has received any special training in caring for these residents.

Facilities where dementia and alert and oriented residents are comingled, not only on the units, but also as roommates, are not good choices for either population. Such arrangements are rarely successful, as the needs of the dementia residents differ from those of the alert and oriented residents. Incompatibility of both sets of residents leads to frequent hostilities and altercations between them.

Choosing the right facility, one that you are confident will give your loved one good care in a warm and cheerful environment, will go a long way toward easing your anxieties.

Once the patient has been admitted, it is important for the responsible family member to attend and participate in the care planning for the new resident. Most reputable facilities also have a family support group that usually meets once a month and is attended by the facility's social service director.

It is a fact that the more visible the resident's family is at the facility, the better their loved one will be cared for. Most nursing homes will deny this, but it is nevertheless true that keeping an eye on the day-to-day care keeps the caregivers on their toes.

However, it is equally important for visitors to respect and honor the rules, regulations, and schedules of the facility, and not to make unreasonable demands on behalf of themselves or their resident family member. Caregivers at these facilities all have tight schedules of duties and responsibilities, and it is not appropriate for family members of residents to interfere in any way. Nor is it appropriate to criticize or get into altercations with staff. If a visitor has a complaint or concern about caregiving or any other issues, these should be brought to the attention of the SSD, whose job it is to resolve such matters. Families will not endear themselves by throwing their weight around and making a nuisance of themselves at the facility.

On the other hand, family members and friends of the resident can be helpful in volunteering their time and talents to assist during recreation programs. Extra help is always welcome with transporting wheelchair-bound residents and escorting others to and from various programs, assisting in serving snacks, etc. Such help is particularly appreciated during holidays and on other special occasions.

There are two additional issues that should not be overlooked when assessing the quality of long-term care facilities. One of them concerns roommate selection. The other concern is the unreasonable noise level at some facilities. Problems regarding these issues can make a resident's life miserable in what may, in all other respects, be a good facility.

Due to the high cost of private-room occupancy, the majority of nursing home residents share a room with another resident. If your loved one is to share a room, it is essential to ascertain the facility's criteria in selecting roommates.

Matching roommates for compatibility is a challenge in any institution in which a population of diverse individuals is forced to share a room. Nevertheless, efforts must be made not to pair two individuals whose personalities make it obvious that they cannot live in peace in such close proximity. Yet all too often, in too many facilities, this issue is ignored, causing no end of grief for the residents as well as for the caregivers.

As has already been mentioned in chapter 10, in some facilities residents are subjected to unreasonable noise levels generated by near-constant piped-in music, interrupted by staff use of the public address system to page and relay messages to each other throughout the day. Some of the loudspeakers are located just outside and above residents' rooms. Thus, one has to listen to incessant noise of one kind or another. There is never a peaceful moment at these facilities.

Such constant assault on the ears cannot be good for anyone's nervous system, but it is especially detrimental to Alzheimer's residents for whom a peaceful, serene environment is essential. In facilities where the management is sensitive to these needs, such as Magnolia Manor, the public address system is used for emergencies only, and all other communication between staff is conducted by telephone or in person; piped-in music is reserved for mealtime only. Thus, the residents live in a much more peaceful environment.

Last, but by no means least, it is recommended that every resident upon admission to a nursing home provide the facility with a living will that states clearly what the resident wishes to have done for him/her, medically, in the event of a life-threatening crisis. This becomes crucial if a person does not wish to have his or her life prolonged through artificial or heroic interventions. In the absence of a living will, the facility and the patient's physician are required by law to call for the use of any and every means to safeguard the resident's life, regardless of the condition in which a lifesaving procedure may leave him or her.

A living will has to be made by the person to whom it pertains, while he/she is still of sound mind and able to make informed decisions regarding a life-threatening crisis. A living will also makes it easier for the family if the patient is unable to speak for himself or herself. It spares the family from having to make a difficult and painful decision on behalf of a loved one. Most facilities now require such instructions upon admission.

The more we can tell our families about our wishes in the event that we become mentally disabled, the better for all concerned. Most of us put off discussing such issues while we are still in possession of all our mental faculties. We are reluctant even to think about the possibility of becoming mentally incapacitated. Yet it makes so much sense to get our house in order in good time. It will spare our families much grief later, at a time when they may already be distressed by our decline and a health crisis. None of us can know in advance whether or not these measures will ever be needed, and therein lies the dilemma. We don't know, so it makes good sense to be prepared.

In the spirit of "just in case" it should become necessary for my family to place me in a nursing home due to advanced AD or one of the other dementing diseases, I have made up a wish list of measures they can take to reduce my distress and ease my adjustment to the new environment. This is a very personal list. Others may have different preferences and are encouraged to make up their own wish lists. Here is mine:

- Furnish my room with treasures from home so that I will be surrounded and comforted by familiar objects.
- Don't forget framed photos and an album of family pictures.
- Include a small CD player and a selection of my favorite music.
- A couple of plants will brighten my room.
- Special treats will be very much appreciated, such as fresh fruit, a bar of dark chocolate, or even a home-cooked meal (but check with the dietitian of the facility to make sure your selection is on the approved list).
- Take me out for a picnic or a walk. Or, if feasible, bring me home for a holiday meal once in a while.
- Visit me as often as you can. You don't have to stay long.
- Talk to me, even if I can no longer understand everything you tell me.
- Give me hugs, hold my hand, demonstrate your love.
- Don't stop visiting when I no longer recognize who you are. I will still be in need of human interaction and affection. And even though I may not be able to verbalize this to you,

be assured that your continued devotion will not be a waste of your time. It will make me feel better if you continue to be a presence in my life—and you will feel better too.

Alzheimer's patients who are in an advanced stage of the disease are among the most vulnerable of all nursing home residents. They can no longer speak for themselves—they cannot influence the quality of their care. They are our parents and our grandparents, our husbands and our wives, our siblings and our friends. We owe them the most tender loving care we can render them. We must not ignore this responsibility.

Recommended Reading

ALZHEIMER'S ASSOCIATION, Residential Care: A Guide for Choosing a New Home, Alzheimer's Association, Chicago, 1998.

DADDY-BOY, A Family's Struggle with Alzheimer's, Carol Wolfe Konek, Graywolf Press, MN, 1991.

HARD TO FORGET, An Alzheimer's Story, Charles P. Pierce, Random House, New York, 2000.

IN A TANGLED WOOD, An Alzheimer's Journey, Joyce Dyer, Southern Methodist University Press, TX, 1996.

LIVING IN THE LABYRINTH, A Personal Journey Through the Maze of Alzheimer's, Diana Friel McGowin, Elder Books, New York, 1993.

LOSING MY MIND, An Intimate Look at Life with Alzheimer's, Thomas de Baggio, The Free Press, New York, 2002.

MY MOTHER'S DESCENT INTO ALZHEIMER'S: Death in Slow Motion, Eleanor Cooney, Harper Collins, New York, 2003.

SPEAKING OUR MINDS, Personal Reflections from Individuals with Alzheimer's, Lisa Snyder, LCSW, W. H. Freeman & Company, New York, 1999.

THE FORGETTING, ALZHEIMER'S: Portrait of an Epidemic, David Shenk, Doubleday, New York, 2001.

THE 36-HOUR DAY, A Family Guide to Caring for Persons with Alzheimer's Disease, Related Dementing Illnesses, and Memory Loss in Later Life, Nancy L. Mace, et al, The Jons Hopkins University Press, Baltimore, MD, 1981.

THE NEW NURSING HOMES, A 20-Minute Way to Find Great Long-Term Care, Marilyn Rantz, RN, PHD, et al, Fairview Press, Minneapolis MN, 2001.

THE VALIDATION BREAKTHROUGH, Simple Techniques for People with Alzheimer's-Type Dementia, Naomi Feil, MSW, ACSW, Health Professions Press, Baltimore MD, 1993.

WHEN SOMEONE YOU LOVE HAS ALZHEIMER'S, What You Must Know, What You Can Do, What You Should Expect . . ., Marilyn Larkin, Dell Publishing, New York, 1995.

WHEN IT GETS DARK, An Enlightened Reflection on Life with Alzheimer's, Thomas De Baggio, The Free Press, New York, 2003.

YOU FORGOT, BUT I STILL LOVE YOU, REYNOLD, The Alzheimer's Tragedy, Betty Conger, ABC Books, a division of Laura Alexandra Press, Wisconsin Rapids WI, 54494.

VIDEOTAPES

CREATIVE INTERVENTIONS WITH THE ALZHEIMER'S PATIENT, Mary Lucero, Geriatric Resources, Inc., P.O. Box 239, Radium Springs, NM 880054 Phone: 800 359-0390, E-mail: GRI@zianet.com